NEW RESEARCH ON
POSTPARTUM DEPRESSION

NEW RESEARCH ON POSTPARTUM DEPRESSION

ADRIAN I. ROSENFEILD
EDITOR

Nova Science Publishers, Inc.
New York

Copyright © 2007 by Nova Science Publishers, Inc.

All rights reserved. No part of this book may be reproduced, stored in a retrieval system or transmitted in any form or by any means: electronic, electrostatic, magnetic, tape, mechanical photocopying, recording or otherwise without the written permission of the Publisher.

For permission to use material from this book please contact us:
Telephone 631-231-7269; Fax 631-231-8175
Web Site: http://www.novapublishers.com

NOTICE TO THE READER

The Publisher has taken reasonable care in the preparation of this book, but makes no expressed or implied warranty of any kind and assumes no responsibility for any errors or omissions. No liability is assumed for incidental or consequential damages in connection with or arising out of information contained in this book. The Publisher shall not be liable for any special, consequential, or exemplary damages resulting, in whole or in part, from the readers' use of, or reliance upon, this material.

Independent verification should be sought for any data, advice or recommendations contained in this book. In addition, no responsibility is assumed by the publisher for any injury and/or damage to persons or property arising from any methods, products, instructions, ideas or otherwise contained in this publication.

This publication is designed to provide accurate and authoritative information with regard to the subject matter covered herein. It is sold with the clear understanding that the Publisher is not engaged in rendering legal or any other professional services. If legal or any other expert assistance is required, the services of a competent person should be sought. FROM A DECLARATION OF PARTICIPANTS JOINTLY ADOPTED BY A COMMITTEE OF THE AMERICAN BAR ASSOCIATION AND A COMMITTEE OF PUBLISHERS.

LIBRARY OF CONGRESS CATALOGING-IN-PUBLICATION DATA

New research on postpartum depression / Adrian I. Rosenfield, editor.
    p. ; cm.
Includes bibliographical references and index.
ISBN 13 978-1-60021-284-0
ISBN 10 1-60021-284-0
1. Postpartum depression--Research. I. Rosenfield, Adrian I.
[DNLM: 1. Depression, Postpartum. WQ 500 N532 2006]
RG852.N49   2006
618.7'6--dc22   2006018339

Published by Nova Science Publishers, Inc. ✦ New York

CONTENTS

Preface		vii
Chapter I	Psychobiology and Culture in the Development of Postpartum Depression *Bethany A. Sallinen, Allyson A. Gilles and Marie J. Hayes*	1
Chapter II	Postpartum Depression: Latin-American Perspectives *Johann Vega-Dienstmaier and Maria I. Zapata-Vega*	29
Chapter III	Implementing Universal Screening Programmes for Postpartum Depression – Possibilities and Risks *Birgitta Wickberg*	47
Chapter IV	Barriers to Postpartum Depression Screening, Diagnosis and Treatment *Dean A. Seehusen and Gary Clark*	59
Chapter V	Perinatal Depression: Time Course, Symptoms, and Hormones *Alyx Taylor, Vivette Glover and M. Kammerer*	69
Chapter VI	Major Depressive Episode in Postpartum: A Preliminary Prospective 1-Year Naturalistic Follow-Up *Lluïsa Garcia-Esteve, Purificación Navarro-García, Carlos Ascaso Terrén, Jaume Aguado Carné and Anna Torres Giménez*	85
Chapter VII	Postpartum Depression and Childrearing Style on Child Development *Alfonso Pedrós-Roselló*	105
Chapter VIII	A Retrospective Account of Difficulty Coping and Stressors in the First Year Postpartum by First-Time Mothers and Fathers *Stephen Matthey*	121

Chapter IX	Animal Models of Postpartum Depression: Steroid Hormone Contributions and Adult Neurogenesis *Jodi L. Pawluski, Amanda D. Green, Cindy Barha and Liisa AM Galea*	**131**
Chapter X	Utility of the Postpartum Depression Screening Scale among Low-Income Ethnic Minority Women *Rhonda C. Boyd and Heidi Worley*	**151**
Index		**167**

PREFACE

Postpartum depression affects 10-15% of women any time from a month to a year after childbirth. Women with postpartum depression may feel restless, anxious, sad or depressed. They may have feelings of guilt, decreased energy and motivation, and a sense of worthlessness. They may also have sleep difficulties and undergo unexplained weight loss or gain. Some mothers may worry about hurting themselves or their baby. In extremely rare casesless than 1% of new motherswomen may develop something called postpartum psychosis. It usually occurs within the first few weeks after delivery. Symptoms may include refusing to eat, frantic energy, sleep disturbance, paranoia and irrational thoughts. Women with postpartum psychosis usually need to be hospitalized.

Chapter 1 - During the reproductive process, psychophysiological and associated mood states are evolutionarily organized to optimize maternal adjustment and infant care. This chapter will present relevant findings from the animal literature that highlight the importance of considering psychobiological factors in an analysis of maternal motivation, attachment, and responsiveness to the infant. The position to be explored is that neurophysiological events, together with traditional sociocultural practices, are critical for maternal psychological wellbeing during the maternal postbirth transition. Conversely, sources of stress such as infant or maternal illness, psychosocial isolation or disruption exacerbate the risk of postpartal psychological dysfunction.

Risk factors, such as prepartal depression or psychological dysfunction, primiparous status, adverse infant characteristics (e.g. illness, prematurity, difficult temperament, colic), psychosocial stress, and isolation during the postpartum period interact synergistically with the neurophysiological milieu surrounding late pregnancy and parturition. These adverse conditions are frequently created, exacerbated or unaddressed by Western cultural practices surrounding birth and are proposed to play a role in precipitating postnatal psychological dysfunction.

Hence, postpartum depression may be compounded or determined by the delicate interplay of biological and sociocultural influences. Effective and competent maternal functioning, the attachment process and the mother's positive regard of her infant are interdependent processes. Future directions should expand the study of postpartum depression to include the effects of this disorder on the development of the maternal-infant relationship. Our recent work suggests that maternal confidence and perceptions of the infant are linearly eroded by depression symptomatology. The longterm psychological health of both mother and child must be viewed as dynamically interdependent and vulnerable to poor outcome when not properly supported by the psychosocial, sociocultural and neurophysiological climate of the postpartal environment.

Chapter 2 - In the past two decades there has been increasing recognition that mood disorders, particularly depression, are a significant cause of pregnancy-related morbidity. Latin-American researchers have been actively contributing to the field of perinatal psychiatry. This article presents a review of the scientific literature on postpartum depression, available in MEDLINE and LILACS/BIREME databases, developed in Latin-American countries including studies conducted mostly in Brazil, Peru, and Chile. Furthermore, due to the known vast migration of Latin-American individuals into developed countries, selected studies on postpartum depression in women of Latino heritage in the United States of America were also reviewed.

Significant efforts involving the adaptation and validation of widely used instruments for the assessment of postpartum depression in Spanish and Portuguese language, such as the Edinburgh Postnatal Depression Scale, have been reported.

Estimates of the prevalence of depression in puerperal women varied from 5.92% and 48% in different clinical settings. The time at which the maternal assessments were conducted ranged from as early as one day to after up to one year postpartum.

Demographic characteristics, availability of social and financial resources, affective support from partners and family, history of depression and/or other psychiatric symptomatology, other pregnancy-related pathologies, premature births, and neonatal illness, among others, have been consistently identified as associated risk factors for the development of postpartum depression in different studies throughout Latino-America. Similar findings, in addition to migration and acculturation factors, may play a roll in the development of depression in Latino women in the USA.

The impact of perinatal depression in the wellbeing of mothers and their children, and perinatal and pediatric care and beneficial interventions for risk groups such as premature children were addressed in other contributions.

The need for appropriate assessment, diagnosis, and treatment of postpartum depression, and the development of preventive strategies and specific services are discussed.

Chapter 3 - Postpartum depression is the most common complication of childbearing with a prevalence of 10-15%, although there is a wide range of rates in different countries. The context and consequences of postpartum depression differs from depression during other times, as it may have negative long-term effects not only for the woman and her family, but also the mother–infant relationship and in turn the emotional and cognitive development of the child. Despite the more or less frequent contacts with health services after childbirth, women with depression often remain undiagnosed and untreated. Reliable, valid screening instruments have, however, been developed and psychological, as well as pharmacological, interventions, have demonstrated to be effective. As a consequence, screening programmes for postpartum depression have been introduced in primary health care services in several countries. Along with these approaches, the evidence base and the possibilities and risks of such programmes have been debated, and issues concerning how to best implement service changes in order to improve mental health in the perinatal period are currently being discussed

Chapter 4 - Postpartum depression is the most common psychiatric condition experienced by women during the first year after the birth of a child. Postpartum depression continues to be highly under-recognized and under-treated despite a recent increase in public and professional interest. There are many barriers to proper screening, diagnosis and treatment that help to explain this trend. Patient barriers include a lack of knowledge about constitutes "normal" feelings in the postpartum period, a lack of knowledge about where to turn for help, fear of stigmatization and fear of using antidepressant treatment while breastfeeding. Provides barriers include a lack of knowledge about the frequency or severity of postpartum depression, a lack of knowledge that validated screening tools exist, uncertainty about how to treat identified women, fear of prescribing antidepressants to lactating women, a lack of time to screen and diagnose, and a lack of financial compensation for diagnosis and treatment. Recent research has looked at these barriers and suggests possible ways of overcoming them.

Chapter 5 - There is growing evidence that perinatal depression does not arise and develop in the same way for all women. We show here examples of how, for some, the symptoms start in pregnancy and resolve postpartum. For other women the symptoms are triggered by parturition itself. In a third group women experience a constant level of symptoms throughout. To enable research into the biochemical basis for these differences, the subtypes must be identified.

There is a large rise in plasma oestrogen, progesterone, corticotropic releasing hormone (CRH), and cortisol levels during pregnancy; cortisol, in late gestation, reaches levels found in Cushing's syndrome and major melancholic depression. Upon parturition levels of all these hormones decrease rapidly. Cortisol, oestrogen and progesterone all have strong psychoactive effects, and their sudden withdrawal may contribute to mood changes. It is possible that depression that starts in pregnancy more closely resembles the melancholic type associated with hypercortisolaemia, while depression that arises postpartum shows more of the symptomatology and hypocortisolaemia of the atypical type. Some women experience mild bipolar II depression postpartum, a subtype also associated with atypical symptoms. Different putative factors (genetic, hormonal and social) probably play a greater or lesser part in the etiology of postnatal depression in different women. It is important to distinguish time of onset and resolution of perinatal affective disorder when investigating causal factors and symptom profile.

Chapter 6 - Objective: This study examined the 12-month clinical course of major depressive episodes (MDE) in postpartum.

Method: Prospective, naturalistic, longitudinal study with a cohort of 140 women. All subjects were assessed at baseline with the Structured Clinical Interview (SCI) according to DSM-IV criteria for major depressive episode. Follow-up was performed at two, six, twelve, eighteen and twenty-four months using the Longitudinal Interval Follow-up Evaluation (LIFE-UP), to obtain information prospectively on syndrome and overall illness severity and treatment. Kaplan-Meier curves were constructed to assess the likelihood of partial and full remission.

Results: The average follow-up time of the cohort was 41.9 weeks (range: 1-52 weeks). 89.3 % of cohorts completed the 2-month follow-up, while 76.4 % reached the 1-year follow-up. At six-month follow-up, 71,4% (95% CI: 62-78,6%) of women reached, at least, partial remission, while 41,4% (95% CI: 31,8-49,7) achieved full remission. After 1-year follow-up 87,6% (95% CI:79,5-92,5) reached partial and 64% (95% CI: 54-72%) full remission. The median time until partial remission was 16 weeks (95% CI: 13-19 weeks) and 32 weeks (95% CI: 25.5-38.5 weeks) in the case of full remission.

Conclusion: The MDE in postpartum context is not a benign or a transient disorder. Postpartum is not a protective context with respect to prognosis of major depression in mothers. The knowledge that almost a third of mothers with a major depressive episode didn't reach full recovery at 1 year of follow-up may help to refine the guidelines of depression diagnosis and treatment during pregnancy and postpartum.

Chapter 7 - Introduction: There are studies which describe association between postpartum depression and child development, but they lack methodological uniformity. In this work we study the influence of the postpartum depression on child development during the first twenty-eight months of life. We study also the childrearing style of the mother, as the possible mediator of the relationship between postpartum depression and child development.

Methods: It is a longitudinal and prospective study including 205 primipara mothers and their children. The definitive sample includes 23 depressed women and 37 women belonging to the control group. The assessments were carried out independently and blindly at the third day after the delivery and at the 1st, 3rd, 6th, 12th and 28th months. The clinical assessment of the mother was made through a clinical interview, the Present State Examination, and a scale of social adaptation. The childrearing received by the mother during her childhood and adolescence was assessed through the Perceived Childrearing Assesment Questionaire, based on the Parental Bonding Instrument developed by Parker. The childrearing received by the children was studied through an instrument based on the direct observation at home of the interaction between the mother and her child at varied ecologic circumstances. Two aspects of the interaction mother-child were assessed: 'affection' and 'care'. The development of the children was assessed using Barley scales of infant development. It was also studied the social development using Stein scale.

Results: A 13.5 % of the women studied have postpartum depression. There are not significant differences regarding perceived childrearing between depressed women and the control group. However, studying the childrearing style of depressed women we observe they bring up their children with a lower level of affection and care than the control group. The length of the depression was determinant in maintaining this lower level of affection and care. During the first year of life, the childrearing style low in affection is associated negatively with the cognitive and social development of the children. At the 28th month the association of a long-course depression and the childrearing style low in affection, during the first year of life, has a negative effect on the cognitive development of the children.

Conclusion: Women with postpartum depression bring up their children with a lower level of affection and care. During the period under study the variable with more weight on the development of the children was a childrearing style low in affection.

Chapter 8 - Much of the work that documents new parents coping experiences is based upon small sample sizes, thus making it difficult to know the rate at which such experiences occur. This study combined qualitative and quantitative information on this issue.

First time parents (221 mothers; 179 fathers) were surveyed one year after the birth about their experiences of coping. Results showed that 24% of women and 10% of men had experienced at least one episode of difficulty coping for more than 2 weeks. For approximately half of these women and men the onset of these longer duration episodes occurred after six weeks postpartum. All mothers and fathers reported that adjusting to the change in their life had impacted on them. In addition, other frequently reported stressors included: baby-care issues and fatigue (mothers and fathers); household chores; infant illness; financial concerns; lack of support; a lack of confidence; and tension with family members (mothers). For men frequent stressors included work-related stress and concern for his partner. There were few differences in reported stressors between women experiencing longer episodes and short episodes of difficulty coping. These data complement the qualitative studies on the experiences of new mothers and fathers, by quantifying the frequency of perceived stressors. This information can be used to normalise the experiences of new parents when providing them with appropriate services. In addition, the data suggest that just screening for psychosocial difficulties at one time point (e.g., 6 weeks postpartum) will miss a considerable proportion of women or men who may have difficulty coping at a later date. The lack of discernible differences in stressors between women self-reporting difficulty coping for long and short durations lends some support to the questionable usefulness of just focusing on women meeting diagnostic criteria for a mood disorder.

Chapter 9 - Postpartum depression (PPD) is a serious medical condition that affects more than 11 % of new mothers. The effects of PPD are debilitating to both the mother and her children. For example, longitudinal studies have revealed that women with untreated PPD have impaired cognitive ability, experience increased marital difficulties, and are more likely to abuse their children, and commit infanticide. In addition, children of mothers with PPD have an increased risk to develop depression or anxiety disorders in adulthood (Nomura et al., 2002), present with impaired cognitive, motor and social development (Murray and Cooper 1997; Nomura et al., 2002) and are less attached to their mothers during infancy (Righetti et al., 2005). The cause of postpartum depression is not known, but PPD and other pregnancy/postpartum-associated neuropsychiatric diseases such as post-partum psychosis have been suggested to be due to the profound hormone fluctuations during pregnancy and the postpartum period (Hendrick et al., 1998). Indeed, estradiol and cortisol/corticosterone are particularly involved in depression and given that there are large fluctuations in these steroid hormones across pregnancy and the post-partum period it may not be surprising that these hormone disturbances are related to the expression of post-partum depression. Furthermore, estradiol and corticosterone have been shown to affect adult neurogenesis in the hippocampus. Adult hippocampal neurogensis is thought to play an important role in depression as chronic antidepressants upregulate hippocampal neurogenesis (Malberg et al., 2000), and animal models of depression show suppressed levels of neurogenesis (Jaako-Movits and Zharkovsky, 2005; Jayatissa, et al., 2006). The present review will focus on the role of the steroid hormones, estradiol and corticosterone, in the development and treatment of PPD, focusing on animal models of PPD which we have previously described and are presently developing. These animal models are based on estrogen-withdrawal across parturition (Galea et al., 2001) and elevated corticosterone levels during the postpartum (Brummelte et al, 2006). Understanding the etiology and treatment of this debilitating disorder is essential for determining how we can promote well-being in mothers and their children.

Chapter 10 - Postpartum depression (PPD) is a serious and common mental health problem. Mothers in low-income families have increased rates of depression, but there is limited information available about PPD in ethnic minority groups. The purpose of this pilot investigation was to assess the psychometric properties and appropriateness of the Postpartum Depression Screening Scale (PDSS) in a community sample of low-income, ethnic minority postpartum women. Seventy-six women (89% ethnic minority) were recruited through a community agency and screened in their homes or community centers. The results showed that the PDSS total score had excellent internal consistency and good construct validity. Fifty-six percent of the women scored above the clinical cut-off score on the PDSS. The PDSS demonstrated some utility limitations, however, as issues of literacy, multiple stressors, and large numbers of women scoring above the clinical cut-off were concerns that arose as potential screening problems for postpartum depression within this population.

Chapter I

PSYCHOBIOLOGY AND CULTURE IN THE DEVELOPMENT OF POSTPARTUM DEPRESSION

Bethany A. Sallinen[*], Allyson A. Gilles and Marie J. Hayes
Psychology Department, University of Maine, Orono, ME, USA

ABSTRACT

During the reproductive process, psychophysiological and associated mood states are evolutionarily organized to optimize maternal adjustment and infant care. This chapter will present relevant findings from the animal literature that highlight the importance of considering psychobiological factors in an analysis of maternal motivation, attachment, and responsiveness to the infant. The position to be explored is that neurophysiological events, together with traditional sociocultural practices, are critical for maternal psychological wellbeing during the maternal postbirth transition. Conversely, sources of stress such as infant or maternal illness, psychosocial isolation or disruption exacerbate the risk of postpartal psychological dysfunction.

Risk factors, such as prepartal depression or psychological dysfunction, primiparous status, adverse infant characteristics (e.g. illness, prematurity, difficult temperament, colic), psychosocial stress, and isolation during the postpartum period interact synergistically with the neurophysiological milieu surrounding late pregnancy and parturition. These adverse conditions are frequently created, exacerbated or unaddressed by Western cultural practices surrounding birth and are proposed to play a role in precipitating postnatal psychological dysfunction.

Hence, postpartum depression may be compounded or determined by the delicate interplay of biological and sociocultural influences. Effective and competent maternal functioning, the attachment process and the mother's positive regard of her infant are

---

[*] Correspondence concerning this article should be addressed to Bethany Sallinen, Psychology Department 5742 Little Hall University of Maine. Orono, Maine 04469. Tel: 207-581-2039; Fax: 207-581-6128; E-mail: Bethany.Sallinen@umit.maine.edu.

interdependent processes. Future directions should expand the study of postpartum depression to include the effects of this disorder on the development of the maternal-infant relationship. Our recent work suggests that maternal confidence and perceptions of the infant are linearly eroded by depression symptomatology. The longterm psychological health of both mother and child must be viewed as dynamically interdependent and vulnerable to poor outcome when not properly supported by the psychosocial, sociocultural and neurophysiological climate of the postpartal environment.

During the reproductive process, psychophysiological and associated mood states are evolutionarily organized to optimize maternal adjustment and infant care. This chapter will present relevant findings from the animal literature that highlight the importance of considering psychobiological factors in an analysis of maternal motivation, attachment, and responsiveness to the infant. The position to be explored is that neurophysiological events, together with traditional sociocultural practices, are critical for maternal psychological wellbeing during the maternal postbirth transition. Conversely, sources of stress such as infant or maternal illness, psychosocial isolation or disruption exacerbate the risk of postpartal psychological dysfunction.

Postpartum depression phenomena and issues related to its measurement as well as psychobiological and sociocultural events and how they relate to recent changes in Western societies are reviewed. These linkages may provide some insight into the observation that the peripartal period is problematic for mood regulation in some women.

ETIOLOGY

The weeks or months following birth represent a psychologically vulnerable period for women (Kendell, McGuire, & Connor, 1981; O'Hara, Rehm & Campbell, 1982; Hopkins, Marcus & Campbell, 1984; O'Hara, Zekoski, Philips, & Wright, 1990). Psychological symptoms of postpartum depression range from mild to severe and are typically affective in nature (Inwood, 1985; Whiffen, 1992; Whiffen & Gotlib, 1993). Current estimates of incidence in the United States and Great Britain are different for each subtype of postpartum depression (O'Hara, 1986; Gotlib, Whiffen, Mount, Milne, & Cordy, 1989; O'Hara et al., 1990); but there is an inverse relationship between incidence and severity suggesting that some postpartum crises may be etiologically distinct (Nott, 1987). There is considerable confusion about the various forms of postpartum psychological dysfunction.

A UNIQUE DIAGNOSIS?

Extensive investigation of postpartum depression in the past decade and a half has lead to controversy regarding its validity as a distinct form of affective disorder (Whiffen and Gotlib, 1993). Those who oppose distinguishing postpartum depression from unipolar depression argue that the clinical presentation, prevalence, course, duration, and etiology of this form of maternal depression during the postpartum period are not distinct from those observed in depression seen at other times (Watson, Elliot, Rugg, & Brough, 1984; Whiffen, 1992; Whiffen & Gotlib, 1993). Whiffen (1992) has argued that the imposition of an artificial distinction between postpartum and nonpostpartum depression has confused this research area, and hampered the treatment of women who become depressed after the birth of a child.

While postpartum depression may be qualitatively similar to unipolar depression on several of the dimensions noted above, there are important problems of identification with regard to the overlap of depressive symptomatology and the normal somatic symptoms of the perinatal period. Studies that rely on self-report symptom checklists to assess depression in the postpartum period often lead to higher rates of self-reported depression, due to the inclusion of questions about fatigue, eating, sleeping, and other somatic changes that are quite normal during the reproductive process. For example, Whiffen (1991) found that Beck's Depression Inventory (BDI) was not sensitive to postnatal depression and resulted in one-third false negatives. Hence, these measurement inconsistencies play an important role in estimating prevalence and in distinguishing mood dysphoria from clinical status.

To address this issue, instruments have been designed specifically for the assessment of depression during the postnatal period (Whiffen, 1991). In one investigation of postpartum depression, Campbell and Cohn (1991) used the Center of Epidemiological Studies-Depression (CES-D) scale which includes fewer somatic symptoms than the BDI, and a modified and shortened version of the Schedule for Affective Disorders and Schizophrenia. Depression was diagnosed using a modification of the Research Diagnostic Criteria (RDC). A semistructured interview was also used in which women were asked about their mood during the postpartum period and about the major symptoms of depression. The questions addressed the duration of the depressed mood and whether women were currently depressed. The frequency with which depressed and nondepressed women reported both somatic and cognitive or affective symptoms of depression was examined. In the nondepressed group, 39% of the women endorsed at least one somatic symptom. By contrast, each cognitive or affective symptom was reported by fewer than 10% of nondepressed women.

Cox, Murray and Chapman (1993) examined this issue further in a two-stage screening procedure using the Edinburgh Postnatal Depression Scale (EPDS), which assessed the intensity of depressive symptoms present within the previous seven days, and Goldberg's Standardized Psychiatric Interview. Two hundred-thirty-two women who were neither pregnant nor had a baby in the previous 12 months were compared six months after delivery and matched for age, marital status, and number of children. Additionally, the 28-item General Health Questionnaire was used, which has four subscales of seven items each: somatic symptoms, anxiety and insomnia, social dysfunction, and severe depression. The presence of defined psychiatric symptoms within the previous seven days and six months, as well as the duration and intensity, and time of onset of depression were assessed. No significant difference in the point prevalence of depressive symptomatology at six months was found between the postnatal (9.1%) and control women (8.2%), but a threefold higher rate of onset of depressive symptoms was found within five weeks of childbirth. The results of this study confirm earlier studies that have suggested that the prevalence of depression in postnatal women is similar to that found in the general population of reproductive aged women.

Such results highlight two important specifications for using the EPDS in different populations. Validation studies suggest that when the EPDS is applied to the general population, the positive predictive value for postpartum depression is less than 50% due to the high proportion of false positives, compared to its use in a clinical setting (Eberhard-Gran, Eskild, Tambs, Opjordsmoen, & Samuelsen, 2001). This finding emphasizes the importance of clinical verification of the diagnosis. However, the finding of an increased risk of such depressive symptoms commencing shortly after delivery suggests that childbirth and its immediate psychosocial sequelae are likely to be important causal factors for non-psychotic depression.

In the next sections potential mechanisms for the increased risk for compromised psychological functioning in the postpartal period will be explored. First, we will examine the cascade of physiological and neurophysiological events that occur during pregnancy, parturition and lactation and propose that, under optimal conditions, these events enhance the expression of adaptive maternal responsiveness. However, in a small percentage of women these neurophysiological conditions may become dysregulated by genetic, illness-related or environmental stress. Second, we will describe the critical role of levity and support from the social environment during the reproductive process which may be less available in modern societies. Because psychological vulnerability is high during this transition period, psychobiological factors may require certain environmental prerequisites to operate adaptively.

MATERNAL RESPONSIVENESS

In this section, evidence will be presented that goes beyond a traditional model of postpartum depression which argued that postpartum events are mediated by endocrine imbalance(s) (Dalton, 1971). Recent examinations of the endocrine argument have improved on the scientific rigor which was weak in the original work and will be discussed in a later section (review: Bloch, Daly & Rubinow, 2003). The argument proposed herein is that postpartum depression is a complex phenomenon whose risk may be related to a significant extent to the failure of the environment to provide critical support to the mother during the reproductive process for fostering the maternal-infant bond, and adequate instrumental and psychological relief to maximize the rate of physical recovery during the postbirth period.

Like other mammals, important evolutionary mechanisms are suggested to be operative in human mothers that potentiate maternal responsiveness to offspring by altering the CNS-mediated maternal motivational state and associated sensory reactivity to infants during the perinatal period. The theoretical basis of this position relies on the animal psychobiology literature concerning maternal motivation, adjustment and responsiveness during the perinatal period in mammalian species (Krasnegor & Bridges, 1990; for a review see Russell, Douglas, & Ingram, 2001). Carefully timed endogenous psychophysiological events during reproduction interact synergistically with sociocultural and psychosocial factors. Hence, the environmental milieu may support, neglect or derail the mother's transition from pregnancy to effective postnatal parenting and resumption of family and work roles. It is proposed that both acute postpartum psychosis and clinical postpartum depression may be triggered by single or multi-tiered disruption of the delicate postpartal adjustment process.

Under optimal conditions the physiological and labor-related events of late pregnancy, parturition and the immediate post-birth period represent a critical zone sculpted by evolution to potentiate and facilitate maternality and thereby insure the survival of the neonate (Corter & Fleming, 1990; Trivers, 1972; Daly & Wilson, 1988). It is critical for the establishment of the maternal-infant bond in mammals that the mother express a strong psychological commitment to infant caretaking, lactation and protection. Maternal protectiveness in animal studies has included aggression towards any threat to the offspring (Ostermeyer, 1983; Svare, 1981).

Neuroendocrine-Behavior Mechanisms in Animal Maternality

Findings in animal psychobiology have suggested potentially important links between mammalian and human maternal responsivity. The psychobiological approach emphasizes the interplay between physiological timing, appropriate sensory stimulation from the infant and maternal motivation and postbirth adjustment (Fleming & Blass, 1994; Rosenblatt, 1965). Findings in mammalian species have established that the mother's neuroendocrine status at the end of pregnancy and following birth induces short-latency maternal responsiveness (Bridges, 1977; Siegel & Rosenblatt, 1975). Further, disruption of pre- and post-parturitional physiological events can lead to maladaptive behavior, including infant rejection and infanticide (Kinsley & Bridges, 1986).

The successful engagement of maternal behavior in the immediate postpartum period is critical to the survival of the neonate in altricial (developmentally immature) mammalian species which include humans. Mammalian and primate mother-infant pairs in the immediate postpartum period express a significant range of maternal responsiveness which varies in competence (Harlow, Harlow, & Hansen, 1963). One factor mediating competence is neurophysiological status. For example, in sheep and in mammalian species including humans the hormonal climate at parturition is characterized by rising estrogen in a background of high, but falling, progesterone levels (Keverne, 1988). Post-birth, this precipitous decline in progesterone continues, and within several hours of birth, estrogen levels decline rapidly as well. In rats, the hormonal climate can be experimentally arranged to simulate birth. Such studies have found that estrogen and, under some conditions, prolactin, facilitate and/or induce maternal behavior in nonpregnant females and neonatally castrated males (the latter procedure is a permanent CNS "feminizing" procedure due to the absence of neonatal testosterone) (Siegel & Rosenblatt, 1975). Oxytocin also increases dramatically during labor in a variety of species (Chard, Hudson, Edwards, & Boyd, 1971) and in estrogen-primed, ovariectomized female rats induces short-latency maternal behavior (Pedersen & Prange, 1979).

Prolactin secretion is stimulated by high estrogen levels associated with the birth process and continues to be secreted at high levels during lactation. In rats, prolactin has been shown to correlate with maternal protective aggression in the early lactational period when titres are highest. However, infants must be suckling for maternal aggression to occur.

Pharmacological evidence suggests that it is high serotonin turnover in the hypothalamus during suckling, in concert with opioid release, that enhances the expression of maternal aggression (Ieni & Thurmond, 1985; Kinsley & Bridges, 1986). In animals, the maintenance of maternal responsiveness and maternal aggression is determined by maternal experience with the offspring. Rosenblatt and colleagues have established that the rat mother is less disrupted in her maternal responsiveness if she has had several days of interaction with the pups before the offspring are removed for 4-5 days after birth (Doerr, Siegal, & Rosenblatt, 1981).

It is known that the role of endocrinology in the induction of maternal behaviors is not as straightforward in primates. Estrogen stimulates progressive increases of cortisol throughout pregnancy in squirrel monkey females (Coe, Murai, Weiener, Levine, & Siiteri, 1986), and there is a marked rise in ACTH (adrenocorticotrophic hormone) and endorphins (Goodlin & Sackett, 1983). Similar changes in the pituitary adrenal axis occur in humans. Cortisol levels rise 3-4 times the normal level during gestation, peaks and quickly declines following parturition (Smith & Thompson, 1991). CRH (corticotrophic releasing hormone) and beta-endorphin both rise with gestational age (Brinsmead, Smith, Singh, Lewin & Owens, 1985). CRH is produced in large amounts amounts by the placenta, rising rapidly from 50 pg/ml at 28 weeks to over 1400 pg/ml at birth (Campbell et al., 1987). Thyroid function is stimulated during pregnancy by placenta-produced human chorionic gonadotropin (Glinoer et al., 1990). However, no maternal priming role has been identified for any specific hormone in primates although brain lesions in the limbic system and olfactory system can disrupt maternal care (Stecklis & Kling, 1985).

Neuroendocrine-Behavior Mechanisms in Human Maternality

Following birth, human mothers typically are quite solicitous of the needs of the newborn (Klaus & Kennel, 1970). If the mother breastfeeds, the intense, physical connection between the mother and the infant continues for a significant period beyond pregnancy. Infant cues (e.g., crying, fussing, motor activity, appearance) are effective elicitors of caretaking and milk letdown (Daly & Wilson, 1988; Fleming, Steiner & Anderson, 1987).

Infant stimulation and caretaking can be elicited in nonmaternal females by several days of exposure to infant olfactory and somatosensory cues. This phase of "maternal" responsiveness is experience-mediated. In human mothers, recognition and attraction to their own infant's odors from worn undershirts has been found after brief postbirth bonding time with their infants (Porter & Schaal, 1991). Maternal feelings of attachment to the infant correlate positively with the time of initial holding (> 15 minutes) in the perinatal period, a condition which creates a flood of infant sensory cues (Troy, 1995).

Although there is little direct evidence for a role of maternal hormones in the facilitation or induction of maternal responsivity in humans some interesting leads have emerged. For example, two interesting candidates, cortisol and hypothalamic pituitary axis peptides such as CRH that rise during pregnancy remain high for several days into the post-birth period in primates and humans (Jolivet, Blanchier, Gautray, & Dhem, 1974; Lowry, 1993). The rapid rise in maternal CRH, ACTH and cortisol levels during pregnancy may interact with prenatal stress to augment the incidence of premature labor, delivery and low birth weight (Sandman, Wadha, Chica-Demet, Dunkel-Schetter & Porto, 1997; McLean, Thompson, Zhang, Brinsmead, & Smith, 1994). Further, CRH levels in the third trimester correlate with length of gestation (Wadwa, Porto, Garite, Chicz-DeMet and Sandman, 1998).

Fleming et al. (1987) examined the dynamic range of cortisol during pregnancy and parturition in women 2-3 days following birth, and found heightened attachment responses in women with higher cortisol levels (r = 0.53). Fleming, Ruble, and Flett (1990) has argued that the heightened state of arousal of new mothers, perhaps, mediated by elevated cortisol, may increase sensitivity to infant cues. However, pregnancy and parturition levels of cortisol may overstimulate arousal mechanisms in some women. Such conditions could enhance mood instability in the postpartum period (Brinsmead et al., 1985). One consequence could be compromised or negative responses to the infant.

CNS Restructuring and Maternal Response

Much effort has been devoted in recent years to searching for the part of the brain that mediates maternal responsiveness. A small cluster of neuronal cells in the medial preoptic area of the female hypothalamus (a structure in the forebrain implicated in reproductive behaviors) responds to estrogen stimulation by inducing dramatic, short latency, maternal responsiveness in nonpregnant female rats (Fahrbach & Pfaff, 1986; Numan, Rosenblatt, & Komisauruk, 1977; Numan & Numan, 1996). The preoptic area and associated circuitry in the limbic system and brainstem can activate maternal drive state in animals.

Maternal motivation and behavior as a psychological construct appears to be primed by the unique hormonal events of late pregnancy, birth and lactation and is activated by infant sensory cues. Fleming, Suh, Korsmit, and Rusak (1994) found an increase in Fos-like immunoreactivity in the medial preoptic area and limbic structures following maternal-pup interactions. The implication of these findings is that experience with the offspring in combination with neuroendocrine priming of the CNS activates genetic events that result in neuronal plasticity.

The role of dopamine, an important neurochemical system involved in arousal modulation and motivation, may play a role in maternal responsiveness and human postpartum depression (see Psychobiology and Postpartum Depression below). Fleming, Korsmit and Deller (1994) found that postpartum rat mothers or nulliparous rats that had been induced to become maternal by hormones or extended infant exposure would work to produce infant stimulation more than control animals. When postpartum animals received a dopamine antagonist this preference was abolished. As was found in human studies of the neurochemical correlates of postpartum depression (Marks, Wieck, Checkley, & Kumar, 1991; McIvor et al., 1996), dopamine regulation may play a role in facilitating psychological stability and adaptation to the postbirth demands of infant care.

The dysregulation of hypothalamic pituitary axis secretion during pregnancy may continue in the postpartal period. Although cortisol does not differentiate postpartum depressed from nondepressed women (O'Hara, Schlechte, Lewis, & Varner, 1991; Abou-Saleh, Ghubash, Karim, Krymski, M., & Bhai, I, 1998), chronic stress during pregnancy may cause a precocious rise in the normal developmental changes during pregnancy in HPA axis activity (Sandman et al., 1997). A dysregulated or more rapid decline in postpartal cortisol levels may result. These changes may mediate disinterest or lower responsiveness to the infant postpartally as Fleming et al. (1984) observed in women with lower cortisol. Lower maternal responsiveness is often seen in postpartum depression. The role of psychosocial stress which has been reliably associated with depression in pregnant and postpartal women will be discussed further in later sections.

In the animal literature, oxytocin has been found to facilitate many events besides uterine contractions during labor and milk ejection. One is to stimulate growth of synaptic connections in the preoptic area of the hypothalamus during the lactational postpartum period (Hatton & Tweedle, 1982; Perlmutter, Tweedle, & Hatton, 1984). Some of this neuronal outgrowth regresses following weaning of the offspring but some changes are permanent. This finding is the first evidence for a neurostructural basis for maternal competencies related to parity. The proposed mechanism is one of enduring neural plasticity produced by peptide secretion during the peripartal period. Recently, it has been argued that one reason infant mortality is higher among the offspring of teenage mothers is due to low maternal competence which may in turn be influenced by immature neurophysiological responsiveness and decreased readiness for reproduction and parental care (Warren & Shortle, 1990; Apter, Viinikka & Wihko, 1978).

PSYCHOBIOLOGY AND POSTPARTUM DEPRESSION

The proposed model between women's biology and their postpartal psychological distress links psychological dysfunction and the physiological challenge of late pregnancy and parturition. Attempts to relate levels of estrogen, progesterone, thyroid hormones, prolactin and other neurochemical products to the appearance or severity of dysphoric symptoms have not yielded positive findings for the most part. One source of confusion is that most studies have been methodologically flawed by inadequate sample size and inappropriate controls (Nott, Franklin, Armitage, & Gelder, 1976; Handley, Dunn, Waldron, & Baker, 1980; Susman & Katz, 1988). For example, Dalton (1989) reported that daily progesterone treatment, administered to counteract the precipitous decline in progesterone following delivery, reduced recurrent postpartum depression to 7% compared to 67% in untreated controls. However, this study is flawed by the absence of a placebo treatment group, suggesting both subject and experimenter bias.

In a separate investigation, Wieck et al. (1991) examined whether recurrent postpartum psychosis was predicted based on the mothers' dopaminergic response to the postbirth decline in estrogen levels. A hormone challenge test of small doses of apomorphine, a dopamine agonist, was given 4 days after delivery. Fifty percent of the treated subjects who were at-risk for recurrent postpartum disorder responded to the apomorphine challenge with dysphoric symptoms but none of the untreated at-risk or control subjects did.

In a follow-up study from the same group, McIvor et al. (1996) tested the responsiveness of dopamine neurons during the postpartum period in women with a history of major depression. On day 4 postpartum before any had relapsed, 14 women were evaluated for dopamine (D2) receptor status by injections of apomorphine. Women who later relapsed with major depression, anxiety and panic disorders had significantly greater dopamine sensitivity as indexed by higher growth hormone levels following apomorphine.

These findings are interpreted as evidence for dopamine supersensitivity in vulnerable individuals due to rapidly lowered estradiol at delivery and suggest a biochemical mechanism mediating mood lability at this time. Estradiol is known to downregulate the 5-HT autoreceptor and upregulate tryptophan hydoxylase leading to increased serotonergic function (Pecins-Thompson & Bethea, 1999). Progesterone withdrawal in the immediate postpartum period reduces GABAergic inhibitory activity (Paul & Purdy, 1992). These neurotransmitter systems are known to mediate, respectively, mood and anxiety.

Thyroid dysfunction may be a sequelae of the rigors of pregnancy as 40% of women had abnormally high levels at 6 weeks postpartum and 5% developed thyroid abnormalities (Walfish, Meyerson, Provias, Vargas, & Papsin, 1992). Postpartum depression was identified in 38% of a sample of women who developed postpartum thyroid disorders which was resolved with thyroid treatment (Pop et al., 1991).

Neuropsychological sensitivity to the tremendous number and pattern of neuroendocrine changes during pregnancy and parturition may be a individual characteristic increasing risk. Links relating risk for postpartum depression, premenstrual syndrome, menopausal symptomatology and sensitivity to oral contraceptives suggests that reproductive hormones may produce mood dysregulation in vulnerable individuals (Block et al., 2003).

Parity, Past Attachment Relationships, and Postpartum Depression

The effects of parity on maternal competence have been demonstrated in many species. Parity is a unique factor in that its effects are clearly experience-based, but is known to have neurophysiological consequences which have been recently demonstrated. The parity effect is mediated by CNS restructuring from previous cycles of reproductive hormone exposure or from experiencing parturition itself (Gibber, 1986; Bridges, 1977; Moltz & Kilpatrick, 1980). During parturition in sheep, sensory stimulation of the cervix (the analogue of fetus expulsion) in combination with estradiol and progesterone priming induces maternal behavior in 80% of nonpregnant female ewes (Keverne, Levy, Poindrum, & Lindsay, 1983). Sensory blockade via peridural anaesthesia during labor significantly delayed maternal behavior onset in primiparous ewes, but only in 25% of multiparous sheep. These effects were not due to the nonspecific effects of paralysis. Early exposure to infants may function to improve psychological adjustment to the neonate. In mammalian species, the multiparous female is more maternal, responds with a shorter latency and is less likely to ignore or kill the offspring, than females with no previous reproductive experience (primates: Montagu, 1981; rodents: Rosenblatt, 1965; DeVries, 1987).

Despite the relationship between parity and maternality in animals, there is little clear evidence for a role for parity in postpartum depression risk. However, many studies have primarily focused on primiparous samples (e.g. Kumar & Robson, 1984). Although increased risk has been reported in both primiparous women (Gard, Handley, Parsons & Waldron, 1986) and multiparous women (O'Hara, 1986; Alfonso, Mayberry & Sheptak, 1988; Shoeb &

Hassan, 1990) the psychobiological role of reproductive experience in maternal functioning is not clear.

In a Danish register study of first psychiatric admission for first episode psychosis within one year after parturition, Videbech and Gouliaev (1995) found that of the women in their sample (N=632), 58% were primiparous, as compared to 44% of the control group. The effect of parity on disease risk was mostly seen among women 25 years of age or older. However, if the patients admitted after the first month postpartum are excluded, the frequency of primiparae in the sample was increased to 82%. In this study the postpartum period was associated with increased risk: admission within one month of delivery accounted for 44% of all of the admissions, the remainder of cases was evenly distributed over the following 11 postpartal months. In another study, Beeghly et al. (2002) report that as a whole primiparous mothers' average CES-D scores in their sample were at their highest levels of depressive symptomatology at two months, and that these mothers were at increased risk for elevated levels across the first year post birth.

Prior experience with infants and children in facilitating maternal adjustment to the infant has been studied to some extent. Fleming et al. (1990) found that maternal attitude during pregnancy predicts postpartum maternality, and is influenced by attachment history and experience with infants. Prior experience with children and attachment to one's mother and husband/partner were important protective factors in predicting the occurrence of postpartum depression. In another longitudinal study, Fleming found that mothers' mood states were most affected by prior experience with infants, and mood was the best predictor of maternal attitude.

Attachment experiences during infancy and early childhood are believed to qualitatively affect one's ability to establish intimacy, a recognized prerequisite for social commitment in adulthood, including relationships with one's offspring. In humans, orphanage rearing and unstable foster-care represent complex socioemotional environments in which long term, intimate care giver attachments often do not occur. Individuals raised under these conditions often develop abnormal affective relationships in adulthood (Rutter, 1991). Appropriate early caretaking may function as a preparatory, and perhaps, necessary, component to appropriate parenting responses to infant cues in adulthood.

These findings emphasize the interaction between reproductive processes and risk for postpartum psychosis. One proposition is that some women may experience abnormal neurophysiological events during pregnancy and parturition. This type of dysfunction coupled with genetic vulnerability and/or precipitating stress may set the stage for pupueral psychosis.

Recent advances in the measurement of endocrine and neurochemical events during pregnancy and parturition and improved experimental methods, may shed light on endocrine-behavior relationships in humans (Harris, Parkes, & Phillips, 1992; Harris, Lovett, Newcombe, Read, & Walker, 1994; Wieck et al., 1991). Searching for indirect effects of parturitional hormones on mood regulatory mechanisms is a promising approach and easily conceptualized in relation to the neurophysiology of the peripartal period and maternal motivation.

Genetic Factors in Individual Vulnerability

It is important to note that previous psychiatric history (Paykel, Emms, Fletcher, & Rassaby, 1980; Tod, 1964), previous treatment for emotional problems (Watson et al., 1984), and number of previous depressions (O'Hara et al., 1984; O'Hara et al., 1991) have all been associated with the development of postpartum depression. For example, extent of depressive symptomology during pregnancy is consistently found to be the strongest predictor of postpartum depressive symptomology (O'Hara, Rehm, & Campbell, 1983; O'Hara, Neunaber, & Zekoski, 1984; O'Hara et al., 1991; Pfost, Stevens, & Lum, 1990; Whiffen, 1988). These findings suggest that postpartum depression is a function of the interaction between a pre-existing vulnerability to depression and the physiological and psychological stress associated with childbirth.

MATERNAL WELL-BEING, MATERNAL RESPONSIVENESS AND PERCEPTIONS OF THE INFANT

Maternal perceptions of infant temperament and infant-related stressors are significant factors in the etiology of postpartum depression (Hopkins, Campbell, & Marcus, 1987). Maternal perceptions of infant temperament may be adversely affected by maternal depression, or alternatively, infant behavior may become irritable or "temperamental" in the face of lower maternal responsiveness. Finally, the potential impact of prepartal depression on fetal neuropsychological health is of concern, as it is known that chronic maternal stress (as would be present if the mother were depressed) is adverse for fetal health and reproductive outcome (Sandman et al., 1997; Dipetro et al, 1996).

Temperament as a psychological construct is defined as enduring, neurobiological bias/es in sensory, affective, and cognitive responsiveness that may disrupt or enhance psychological adjustment in various settings (Rothbart, Derryberry, & Posner, 1994; Thomas & Chess, 1977). Research indicates that difficult infant temperament is associated with postpartum depression (Cutrona & Troutman, 1986; Hopkins, Campbell, & Marcus, 1987). Cutrona and Troutman's (1984) mediational model offers an explanation of the link between difficult infant temperament and postpartum depression. The model suggests that difficult infant temperament can increase the risk of maternal depression both directly and indirectly through the mediation of parenting self-efficacy (i.e., low confidence in parenting ability). Thus, this model suggests that a woman's sense of parental competence and overall emotional well-being are related to the temperamental characteristics of her infant.

In a recent study performed in our laboratory, a subset of pregnant women from a multi-phase longitudinal study was examined for symptoms of peripartal depression. The demographics of the sample are representative of disadvantaged families from a large rural area of Northeastern Maine attending a Family Practice Clinic and receiving appropriate prenatal care. Maternal depression was assessed pre- and post- pregnancy using the BDI and EPDSI. Post-pregnancy, mothers completed the Mother and Baby Scale (MABS), which assesses infant temperament and maternal perceptions of caretaking confidence (Wolke & St. James-Roberts, 1987).

We hypothesized that maternal psychological well-being and evidence of postpartum depression would correlate with poor infant adaptation in the postnatal period. Halpern, Anders, & Garcia Coll (1994) and Field et al. (1990) have noted that depressed mothers have infants with more expressions of emotional negativity. This is evidenced by irritability and crying during social interactions with their own mothers and strange mothers. These findings have been interpreted as suggesting that mother-infant interactions are strained in depressed dyads. One possibility is that the infants' emotional needs are not being met in interactions with their depressed mothers. Alternatively, infants share the mother's genetic predisposition toward maladaptation, at least to the extent that maternal mood regulation appears to be influenced by genetic factors.

Our results suggest an association between symptoms of postpartum depression and difficult infant temperament. We compared the EPDS with the factor-analyzed MABS infant dimensions of "Unsettled-Irregular," "Alertness-Responsiveness," and "Easiness," and the maternal dimensions of "Lack of Confidence in Caregiving" and "Global Confidence." High scores on the MABS "Unsettled-Irregular" factor suggest poor regulatory functioning in feeding and sleep, and general infant irritability. Figure 1 illustrates that maternal perceptions of infant temperamental irritability (i.e., "Unsettled-Irregular" factor of the MABS) were correlated with scores of maternal self-reported depressive symptomatology during the postpartal period. Further, as demonstrated in Figure 2, our findings also indicate a moderate association between post-partum depressive symptomatology and maternal ratings of perceived lack of confidence in caregiving. Hence, these preliminary results suggest that maternal mood and infant irritability are intimately linked.

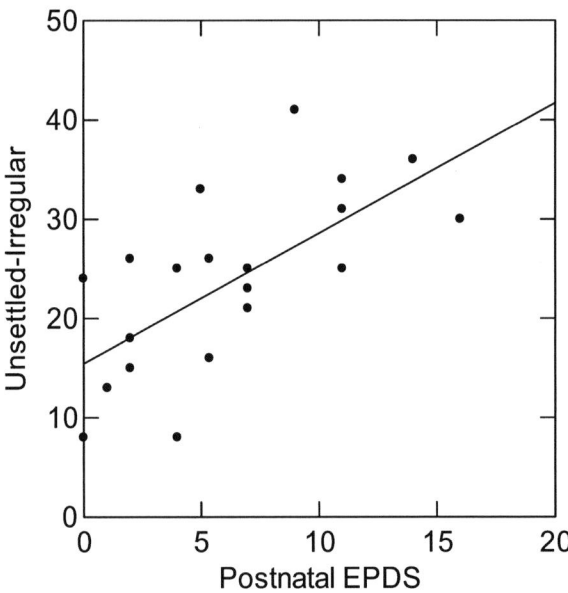

Figure 1. Scatterplot of scores on the Unsettle-Irregular factor of the MABS and postnatal EPDS scores (r = 0.682; p < .001).

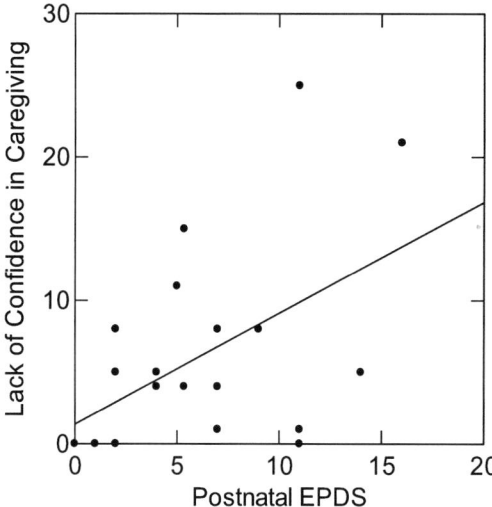

Figure 2. Scatterplot of scores on the Lack of Confidence in Caregiving factor of the MABS and postnatal EPDS scores (r = 0.539; p < .01).

Taken together, these preliminary findings suggest that maternal depression may both exacerbate a difficult infant temperament and contribute to the maintenance of depressive symptoms in the mother. Mother-infant interactions may be a potential mechanism through which these outcomes occur. If depressed mothers are emotionally unresponsive to their infants, a psychobiologically vulnerable infant with a predisposition to an irritable temperament may express this temperamental style in an effort to elicit responsiveness from the mother. It is hypothesized that as a result of the infant's irritability, the mother feels a low level of confidence in her caregiving, and this serves to maintain or enhance her depression. This explanation is consistent with Cutrona and Troutman's (1986) mediational model which suggests that maternal depression in the postpartal period may result from either a difficult infant temperament or low parenting self-efficacy.

CULTURE AND SOCIAL SUPPORT IN POSTPARTUM DEPRESSION

The contribution of culture to situational and/or relational stressors that undermine the unique psychological needs of reproductive women is a poorly studied area, although it is well accepted that the perinatal period is a highly demanding transition period for first-time mothers, as well as women with other children to care for. Nonetheless, several lines of inquiry suggest that postpartum adjustment is perhaps most affected by the social context. In cross cultural studies of non-Western societies, high levels of family and community support are typically activated by childbirth (Jordan, 1980; Tronick, Winn, & Morrelli, 1985; Garcia-Coll, 1989; Muret-Wagstaff, & Moore, 1989). Interestingly, postpartum psychiatric disorders have been rarely reported in non-Western societies although incidence is difficult to interpret in cross cultural studies because of reporting bias and focus on this issue has been limited (Stern & Kruckman, 1983; Egeland & Hostetter, 1983; Bash & Bash-Liechti, 1969).

Oakley (1980) and Ball (1994) have argued that peripartal psychosocial support is lacking in Western societies, particularly in recent times. Correlative rates of maternal psychosis in the first year of the infant's life have been dramatically on the rise in Great Britain in the last thirty years: 0.34/1000 vs. 1.04/1000 (Rehman, St. Clair, & Platz, 1990). Potential contributions to the increase in maternal psychosis may be related to role expectations for mothers in Western society. Western women who have recently given birth are often given insufficient time or assistance for recuperation in the postbirth period before resuming high role expectations (Giovannini, 1992). In the United States and Europe, women are often implicitly expected to independently care for their infant and family almost immediately following birth and are often alone and socially isolated as partners return to work and extended family recedes (Coyne, 1985; Cutrona, 1984; Giovanni, 1992; Oakley, 1980). Although their study did not focused on cross cultural issues, Hopkins, Campbell and Marcus (1987) found that postpartal instrumental support, which is more common in non-Western societies (Chalmers, 1991; LeVine, 1977), was a protective factor for postpartum depression.

In the United States, women who plan to return to work often do not receive adequate maternity leave, particularly paid leave (Friedan, 1986; Hewlett, 1986), although there are notable exceptions in Canada and Scandinavia (Saucier, Bernazzi, Bogeat, & David, 1995). Postbirth instrumental demands, sleep deprivation associated with leaving the bed for night feedings and chronic daytime social isolation set the stage for psychological distress, particularly mood disturbance. The social mobility of modern society creates other culturally-based challenges. Extended families often live quite far from new families who relocate to seek socioeconomic and career-related opportunities. Recent relocation and staying home with the infant disrupts established ecological support networks. Homemakers compared to employed women or women on maternity leave are more likely to be less educated, to experience a lack of psychosocial support, to have an income below the poverty level, to have had an unwanted or mistimed pregnancy, and/or to be placed in situations that are strongly associated with depressive symptomatology in the postbirth period (Richman, Raskins & Gaines, 1991; Des Rivieres-Pigeon, Seguin, Goulet, & Descaries, 2001). Another sociocultural factor is the ideology of motherhood in our society (Rich, 1976). Traditional Western cultural rules or stereotypes of motherhood idealize exclusive care of the infant by the mother despite changing roles for women in our society. Hock and DeMeis (1990) examined the desire to work vs. the desire to stay home with the infant by working and nonworking women who were evaluated immediately postpartum and 12 months later. Women who stayed home with their infants out of a sense of traditional duty, that is, followed a traditional role despite a desire to work, suffered the most depression compared to women who worked and identified strongly with their work role, preferred to remain home and did, or worked out of necessity only. The latter category, women who desired to be home with their infant but were required to work for economic reasons, viewed their work role as an extension of motherhood responsibilities. These results suggest that a serious risk factor for depression in the first 12 months may be role conflict arising from acceptance of the traditional role despite being psychologically uncomfortable with this decision. Ironically, exclusive care of the infant is peculiar to Western culture, whereas most traditional societies share all aspects of infant care among related adults from birth onwards (LeVine, 1977). Richman et al. (1991) argues that the postpartum period is a time of significant psychological risk for husbands/partners as well as mothers. In couples' adjustment to the birth of their infant, middle socioeconomic class, but not lower class partners, showed similar risk for mood disturbance. The authors suggest that middle class couples may be more likely than lower class couples to adopt an egalitarian approach to parenting responsibilities, and more equally share the burden of infant care. Perhaps, as a consequence of new parenting role demands and/or role conflict, middle-class fathers are also at increased risk of developing symptoms of postpartum depression. Similar findings were reported by Atkinson and Rickel (1984) and argue for an ecological basis for postpartum depression.

Most importantly, Western societies may no longer provide a responsive social infrastructure for promoting optimal maternal psychological adjustment in the postbirth phase. Giovannini (1992) theorizes that recent sociocultural trends in Western societies towards the medicalization of childbirth may also interfere with sensitive care of the mother during the postpartum period. Neter, Collins, Lobel, & Dunkel-Schetter (1995) found that dissatisfaction with the labor and delivery process was associated with increased risk for postpartum depression. Other potential sources of culturally-based stress include standard hospital routines that disrupt feeding, social contacts and rest, overly rapid discharge, and overmedication during delivery (Ball, 1994).

Studies examining expectations regarding peripartal medical and psychological support among rural and urban women highlight the importance of cultural norms in understanding potential antecedents of postnatal depression. Rural women, such as those from the Pedi tribe in South Africa and the Beka'a Valley in Lebanon prefer traditional births that include tribal midwives and vaginal delivery rather than Western-style medical attendants and cesarian section (Chaaya et al., 2002). The entire peripartal experience is associated with established cultural practices concerning pregnancy and birth that are holistically related to emotional support and instruction in infant care. In the postpartum period, significant instrumental and psychosocial support is mandated by tradition to be provided by the woman's mother in the Pedi or mother-in-law in the Zulu. Similar levels of parental support are provided to first-time mothers by the parents in the postpartum period in Saudi-Arabia (Shoeb & Hassan, 1990) which may account for lower rates of postpartum depression in primiparous women in this culture.

Immigrant women accustomed to familial and kinship support following childbirth are often at risk for postpartum depression in their non-native environment. Women who traditionally practice cultural rituals that allow for recuperation following childbirth, in which family and friends pamper the new mother with physical and psychological support often experience feelings of loneliness, hopelessness, and being a bad mother if such an experience is not available to them (Nahas & Amasheh, 1999). It is believed that such practices, which are common in countries such as the Middle East, Jamaica, India, and China help to reduce the development of postnatal depression and ameliorate the mood disturbance to a sub-threshold level (Cox, 1999).

Cultural Differences in Psychosocial Stress

Stressors related to pregnancy, childbirth and postpartum adjustment are strongly associated with the expression of postpartum depression in recent studies in the United States, Canada and Europe. This general finding is consistent with the argument that Western society may be unresponsive to the postbirth needs of the recently parturient woman. Heightened levels of postpartum depressive symptomology have been linked to childcare-related stressors (Atkinson & Rickel, 1984; Cutrona, 1984; O'Hara, 1986), pregnancy or delivery complications (Campbell & Cohn, 1991), perceived stress during pregnancy (Gotlib et al., 1991; O'Hara, Rehm, & Campbell, 1982) and post birth (Grazioli & Terry, 2000) and number of stressful life events since delivery (O'Hara, 1986; O'Hara, Schlechte, Lewis, & Verner., 1991). Heightened levels have also been related to delivering an infant preterm (Logsdon & Usui, 2001), at risk for medical problems (Blumberg, 1980), or with difficult temperaments (Hopkins, Campbell & Marcus, 1987). Prospective studies have generally confirmed these variables as antecedents to postpartum depression (Gotlib, Whiffen, Wallace, & Mont, 1991; O'Hara et al., 1991). Neter et al. (1995) evaluated the effects of stress, social support, and labor and delivery experiences on the incidence of postpartum depression in a sample of low-income American women interviewed on several occasions during pregnancy and once at two months postpartum with a focus placed on a range of depressed affect from mild to severe. Variables including prenatal depressive symptoms, satisfaction with paternal and healthcare provider support, chronic stress, state anxiety, financial strain, life events, and satisfaction with labor and delivery were assessed. Postpartum depression was measured using the CESD scale, which maintains a high correlation between it's scores and a diagnosis of depression. The sample was found to be comprised of 67.6% nondepressed respondents and 32.4% depressed respondents. Women experiencing high levels of depressed mood reported less satisfaction with their social support, more prenatal stress, less satisfaction with labor experiences, and less involvement of the infants' father after birth. Respondents with infants that had adverse medical outcomes were more likely to experience postpartum depression.

The sociocultural model predicts that variations in social support availability in Western society may function to protect mothers from postpartum depression. It has been consistently found that friendships, operationally defined by the number of contacts, frequency of contacts, self-report of emotional support, and the quality of relationships including the partner relationship predicts both pre- and postnatal depression (O'Hara, Rehm, & Campbell, 1983; O'Hara 1986; Logsdon, McBride, & Birkimer, 1994; Seguin, Potvin, St. Denis, & Loisell, 1999; Fisher, Feekery, & Rowe-Murray, 2002; Stuchbery, Matthey, & Barnett, 1998). In fact, women suffering from postpartum depression who received partner support are less likely to have a deterioration in their depressive symptomatology and health in general, regardless if the pregnancy is high or low risk (Misri, Kostaras, Fox, & Kostaras, 2000; Besser, Priel, & Wiznitzer, 2002). O'Hara (1986) conducted a prospective longitudinal design in which subjects were administered the Stressful Life Events index and interviewed on several occasions both pre- and post-partum. Postpartum depression was associated with the number of depression episodes in the past, the number of stressful life events after delivery, levels of instrumental support and less social support from parents and parents-in-law.

Further, as the number of children increased so did the risk of depression. Deficient spousal support, characterized by lack of emotion-based talking in combination with poor instrumental support, was identified in the women who developed postpartum depression (Hackel & Ruble, 1991). Other studies have identified marital tension and dissatisfaction both prior to and following the onset of postpartum depression (Ballinger, Kay, & Naylor, 1982; Braverman & Roux, 1978; Cox, Connor, & Kendall, 1982; Gotlib et al., 1991; O'Hara et al., 1983; Watson, Elliot, Rugg, & Brough, 1984). Difficulties within the martial relationship, as well as changes in social support are good predictors of maternal symptoms of depression. Unsupportive marital partners may not only be a source of psychosocial stress within the relationship, but may increase the likelihood that a woman will become more sensitive to the lack of support and breakdown of the relationship. High support need, as well as dissatisfaction with this area of life appears to be a risk factor that increases a woman's vulnerability to postpartum depression due to the inability to cope with partner stressors (Martinez-Schallmoser, Telleen, &MacMullen, 2003; Logsdon, Birkimer, & Usui, 2000). Although the positive effects of a supportive relationship seem to mediate the effects of low postnatal mood, the evidence is not clear as to whether having a conflictual close relationship has more deleterious effects.

Social support has been associated as a mediating factor between mothers' perceived acceptance of early parental relationships and postpartum depressive symptomatology. Crockenberg and Leerkes (2003) found that remembered childhood paternal acceptance was a protective factor for women against postpartum depression when their partners were aggressive. Positive perception of social support and caring relationships may affect maternal well-being, as well as positive perceptions of the newborn (Priel & Besser, 2002). However, the transactional nature of past and current experiences, coupled with the cognitive formation of affective relationships raises the possibility that early relationships may affect subsequent interpersonal relationships, including sensitivity to social support and attachment to the infant ultimately. In a prospective study conducted by O'Hara et al. (1991), vulnerability to depression interacted with life stress to predict 17% of the variance in postpartum depressive symptomology. These studies establish the importance of the social climate and the perception of and satisfaction with social support in easing and maintaining the psychological adjustment of the mother to the myriad of physiological and psychological changes of the postbirth period

The literature suggests a strong relationship among culture, perceived and expected social support, postnatal mood, and maternal attribution style, as reported by Stuchbery, Matthey, and Barnett's (1998) in their examination of postpartum depression among non-English-speaking mothers. Women from cultures who value individual fortitude and self-coping may feel a sense of failure when requiring practical help and emotional support from partners and others, whereas women from cultures whose families share in the child-raising responsibilities may not engage in such self-blame when the need for additional support arises. Maternal cognitions, including feelings of self-efficacy are believed to play an important role in the likelihood of depressive symptoms following childbirth.

Also consistent with previous research and the proposed sociocultural model is that there is less instrumental support in the form of child care aid in Western societies; responsibility for night feedings is typically done by the mother from birth onward. In Japan (Caudill &

Weinstein, 1969), Kenya (Super & Harkness, 1982) and the Mayan peninsula of Mexico (Morelli, Rogoff, & Oppenheim, 1992) mothers and infants co-sleep, which leads to fewer disruptions in the mother's sleep for feedings. Greatly fewer mothers and infants co-sleep in Western compared to non-Western societies (McKenna, Thoman, Anders, Sadeh, Schechtman & Glotzbach, 1993; Hayes, Stowe, & Roberts, 1996) which creates chronic sleep deprivation for women who must awaken and leave their beds for long periods during the night to feed. The cultural practice in Western society of separate sleeping sites for mother and infant carries significant social censure when violated.

CONCLUSION

The reproductive process itself is facilitatory of maternal responsiveness and moderates the stress of labor, delivery and lactation. Neuroendocrine events are critical for the orchestration of peripartal events and amongst other functions serve to reduce the stress of pregnancy (progesterone), pain of delivery (opioids) and transition towards successful lactation (prolactin-mediated reduction in sensory reactivity) (Stern, Goldman, & Levine, 1973). Cortisol in the postbirth period may enhance maternal reactivity to infant cues in the immediate postpartum period (Fleming, Ruble, & Flett, 1990), and potentiate familiarization with the unique odors and somatosensory features of the newborn (Schaal & Porter, 1991).

Maternal readiness and competence in the postpartum period depends on a cascade of carefully timed evolutionary events that are coordinated with sociocultural traditions to ease the transition from pregnancy. Cross-cultural studies of seclusion suggest that the ecology of the birth process and early lactation should ideally utilize a safe and familiar setting without interruptions or demands by the social environment (Stern & Kruckman, 1983). Early and later infant care is greatly assisted by proscribed family members and family concerns are addressed by others on the community. The continuity of the influence of the social environment is supported by the findings that both early experience of adequate affectional bonds with parents (Gotlib et al., 1991), and life experiences with infants and children may ease the acceptance of the infant in both the short and long term. Cutrona and Troutman (1986) have suggested that a psychological state of maternal competence or parental self-efficacy may take some time to develop and may mediate maternal depression especially if the infant is difficult temperamentally. Undoubtedly, familial relationships and cultural practices must coordinate maternal support to maximize the mother's postpartum psychological adjustment.

Risk factors, such as prepartal depression or psychological dysfunction, primiparous status, adverse infant characteristics (e.g. illness, prematurity, difficult temperament, colic), psychosocial stress, and isolation during the postpartum period interact synergistically with the neurophysiological milieu surrounding late pregnancy and parturition. These adverse conditions are frequently created, exacerbated or unaddressed by Western cultural practices surrounding birth and are proposed to play a role in precipitating postnatal psychological dysfunction.

Hence, postpartum depression may be compounded or determined by the delicate interplay of biological and sociocultural influences. Effective and competent maternal functioning, the attachment process and the mother's positive regard of her infant are interdependent processes. Future directions should expand the study of postpartum depression to include the effects of this disorder on the development of the maternal-infant relationship. Our recent work suggests that maternal confidence and perceptions of the infant are linearly eroded by depression symptomatology. The longterm psychological health of both mother and child must be viewed as dynamically interdependent and vulnerable to poor outcome when not properly supported by the psychosocial, sociocultural and neurophysiological climate of the postpartal environment.

REFERENCES

Abou-Saleh, M. T., Ghubash, R., Karim, L., Krymski, M., & Bhai, I. (1998). *Psychoneuroendocrinology, 23*, 465-475.

Alfonso, D. D., Mayberry, L. J., & Sheptak, S. (1988). Multiparity and stressful events. *Journal of Perinatology, 8*, 312-317.

Apter, D., Viinikka, L., & Wihko, R. (1978). Hormonal pattern of adolescent menstrual cycles. *Journal of Clinical Endocrinology and Metabolism, 47*, 944-954.

Atkinson, A. K., & Rickel, A. U. (1984). Postpartum depression in primiparous parents. *Journal of Abnormal Psychology, 93*, 115-119.

Ball, J. A. (1994). *Reactions to Motherhood: The Role of Postnatal Care* (2nd ed.). Great Britain: Cromwell Press.

Ballard, C. J., Davis, R., Cullen, P. C., Mohan, R. N. & Dean, C. (1994). Prevalence of postnatal psychiatric morbidity in mothers and fathers. *British Journal of Psychiatry, 16*, 782-788.

Ballinger, C. B., Kay, D. S. G., & Naylor, G. H. (1982). Some biochemical findings during pregnancy and after delivery in relation to mood change. *Psychological Medicine, 12*, 549-556.

Bash, K.W. & Bash-Liechti, J. (1969). Studies of the epidemiology of neuropsychiatric disorders among the rural population of the province of Khuzestan, Iran. *Social Psychiatry, 4*, 137-143.

Beeghly, M., Weinber, M. K., Olson, K. L., Kernan, H., Riley, J., & Tronick, E. Z. (2002). Stability and change in level of maternal depressive symptomatology during the first postpartum year. *Journal of Affective Disorders, 71*, 169-180.

Besser, A., Priel, B., & Wiznitzer, A. (2002) Childbearing depressive symptomatology in high-risk pregnancies: The roles of working models and social support. *Personal Relationships, 9*, 395-413.

Blumberg, N. L. (1980). Effects of neonatal risk, maternal attitude, and cognitive style on early postpartum adjustment. *Journal of Abnormal Psychology, 89*, 139-150.

Braverman, J., & Roux, J. F. (1978). Screening for the patient at risk for postpartum depression. *Obstetrics and Gynecology, 52*, 731-736.

Bridges, R. S. (1977). Parturition: Its role in the long-term retention of maternal behavior in the rat. *Endocrinology, 114*, 930-940.

Brinsmead, M., Smith, R., Singh, B., Lewin, T. & Owens, P. (1985). Peripartum concentrations of beta endorphin and cortisol and maternal mood states. *Australian and New Zealand Journal of Obstetrical and Gynaecology, 25*, 194-197.

Campbell, S.B., Cohn, J.F., Flanagan, C., Popper, S. & Meyers, T. (1992). Course and correlates of postpartum depression during the transition to parenthood. *Development & Psychopathology, 4*, 9-48.

Campbell, S. B., & Cohn, J. F. (1991). Prevalence and correlates of postpartum depression in first-time mothers. *Journal of Abnormal Psychology, 100*, 594-599.

Campbell, E. A., Linton, E. A., Wolfe, C. D., Scraggs, P. R., Jones, M. T., & Lowry, P. J. (1987). *Journal of Clinical Endocrinology and Metabolism, 64*, 1054-1059.

Caudill, W. & Weinstein, H. (1969). Maternal care and infant behavior in Japan and America. *Psychiatry, 32*, 12-43.

Chalmers, B. (1991). Changing childbirth customs. Pre- and Perinatal Psychology, 5, 221-232.

Chard, T., Hudson, C. N., Edwards, C. R., & Boyd, N. R. (1971). Release of oxytocin and vasopressin by the human fetus during labor. *Nature, 234*, 352-354.

Chaaya, M., Campbell, O.M.R., El Kak, F., Shaar, D., Harb, H., & Kaddour, A. (2002). Postpartum depression: prevalence and determinants in Lebanon. *Archives of Women's Mental Health, 5*, 65-72.

Coe, C. L., Murai, J. T., Weiener, S. G., Levine, S., & Siiteri, P. K. (1986). Rapid cortisol and corticosteroid-binding globulin responses during pregnancy and after estrogen administration in the squirrel monkey. *Endocrinology, 118*, 435-440.

Corter, C. M., & Fleming, A. S. (1990). Maternal responsiveness in humans: Emotional, cognitive, and biological factors. In P. J. B. Slater, J. S. Rosenblatt, & C. Beer (Eds.), *Advances in the Study of Behavior* (Vol. 19, pp. 83-136). New York: Academic Press.

Cox, J.L. (1999). Perinatal mood disorders in a changing culture. A transcultural European and African perspective. *International Review of Psychiatry, 11*, 103-110.

Cox, J. L., Murray, D., & Chapman, G. (1993). A controlled study of the onset, duration, and prevalence of postnatal depression. *British Journal of Psychiatry, 163*, 27-31.

Cox, J., Connor, Y., & Kendall, R. (1982). Prospective study of the psychiatric disorders of childbirth. *British Journal of Psychiatry, 140*, 111-117.

Coyne, J. C. (1985). Strategic therapy with depressed married persons: Initial agenda themes and interventions. *Journal of Marital and Family Therapy, 11*, 337-344.

Crockenberg, S. & Leerkes, E. (2003). Parental acceptance, postpartum depression, and maternal sensitivity: mediating and moderating processes. *Journal of Family Psychology, 17*, 80-93.

Cutrona, C. E. (1983). Causal attributions and perinatal depression. *Journal of Abnormal Psychology, 92*, 161-172.

Cutrona, C. E. (1984). Social support and stress in the transition to parenthood. *Journal of Abnormal Psychology, 93*, 278-390.

Cutrona, C. E., & Troutman, B. R. (1986). Social support, infant temperament, and parenting self-efficacy: A mediational model of postpartum depression. *Child Development, 57*, 1507-1518.

Dalton, K. (1971). Prospective study into puerperal depression. *British Journal of Psychiatry, 118*, 689-692.

Dalton, K. (1989). Successful prophylactic progesterone for idiopathic postnatal depression. *Journal of Prenatal and Perinatal Studies* (pp. 323-327).

Daly, M., & Wilson, M. (1988). The Darwinian psychology of discriminative parental solicitude. *Nebraska Symposium on Motivation, 35*, 91-144.

Dawson, G., Klinger, L. G., Panagiotides, H., Hill, D., & Spicker, S. (1992). Frontal lobe activity and affective behavior of infants of mothers with depressive symptoms. *Child Development, 63*, 725-737.

Dawson, G., Klinger, L. G., Panagiotides, H., Spieker, S., & Frey, K. (1992). Infants of mothers with depressive symptoms: Electroencephalographic and behavioral findings related to attachment status. *Development and psychopathology, 4*, 67-80.

Des Rivieres-Pigeon, C., Seguin, L., Goulet, L., & Descarries, F. (2001) Unravelling the complexities of the relationship between employment status and postpartum depressive symptomatology. *Women & Health, 34*, 61-79.

DeVore, I. (1963). Mother infant relations in free-ranging baboon. In H. L. Rheingold (Ed.), *Maternal behavior in mammals* (pp. 305-333). New York: Wiley.

DiPietro, J. A., Hodgson, D. M., Costigan, K. A., Hilton, S. C. & Johnson, T. R. B. (1996). Fetal neurobehavioral development. *Child Development, 67*, 2553-2567.

Doerr, H. K., Siegel, H. J., & Rosenblatt, J. S. (1981). Effects of progesterone withdrawal and estrogen on maternal behavior in nulliparous rats. *Behavioral and Neural Biology, 32*, 35-44.

Eberhard-Gran, M., Eskild, A., Tambs, K., Opjordsmoen, S., & Samuelsen, S.O. (2001). Review of validation studies of the Edinburgh Postnatal Depression Scale. *Acta Psychiatrica Scandinavica, 104*, 243-249.

Egeland, J.A. & Hostetter, A.M. (1983). Amish study: I. Affective disorders among the Amish, 1976-1980. *American Journal of Psychiatry, 140*, 56-61.

Ehrhardt, A. A., & Baker, S. W. (1974). Fetal androgens, human central nervous system differentiation and behavior sex differences. In R. C. Friedman, R. M. Richard, R. L. Vande Wiele (Eds.), *Sex Differences in Behavior* (pp. 33-51). New York: Wiley.

Fahrbach, S. E., & Pfaff, D. W. (1986). Effect of preoptic region implants of dilute estradiol on the maternal behavior of ovariectomized nulliparous rats. *Hormones and Behavior, 20*, 354-363.

Fisher, J., Feekery, C., & Rowe-Murray, H. (2002). *Journal of Pediatric Child Health, 38*, 140-145.

Fleming, A. S., & Blass, E. M. (1994). Psychobiology of the early mother-young relationship. In J. A. Hogan & J. J. Bolhuis (Ed.), *Causal Mechanisms of Behavioral Development* (pp. 212-241). Cambridge, England: Cambridge Univ. Press.

Fleming, A.S., Korsmit, M., & Deller, M. (1994). Rat pups are potent reinforcers to the maternal animal: Effects of experience, parity, hormones, and dopamine function. *Psychobiology, 22*, 44-53.

Fleming, A. S., Steiner, M., & Anderson, V. (1987). Hormonal and attitudinal correlates of maternal behavior during the early postpartum period in first-time mothers. *Journal of Reproductive and Infant Psychology, 5*, 193-205.

Fleming, A. S., Ruble, D. N., & Flett, G. L. (1990). Adjustment in first-time mothers: Changes in mood and mood content during the early postpartum months. *Developmental Psychology, 26(1)*, 137.

Fleming, A. S., Suh, E. J., Korsmit, M., & Rusak, B. (1994). Activation of Fos-like immunoreactivity in the medial preoptic area and limbic structures by maternal and social interactions in rats. *Behavioral Neuroscience, 108*, 724-734.

Fleming, A. S., & Korsmit, M. (1995). Plasticity in the maternal circuit: Effects of maternal experience on Fos-Lir in hypothalamic, limbic, and cortical structures in the postpartum rat. *Behavioral Neuroscience, 110*, 567-582.

Friedan., B. (1986). *The Second Stage* (rev. ed.) New York: Summit.

Garcia-Coll, C. T. (1989). The consequences of teenage childbearing in traditional Puerto Rican culture. In Nugent, J. K., Lester, B.M. & Brazelton, T.B. (Eds.). *The Cultural Context of Infancy*. (pp.111-132). Norwood, N.J.: Ablex Publishing.

Gard, P. R., Handley, S. L., Parsons, A. D., & Waldron, G. (1986). A multivariate investigation of postpartum mood disturbance. *British Journal of Psychiatry, 148*, 567-575.

Gibber, J. R. (1986). Infant-directed behavior of rhesus monkeys during their first pregnancy and parturition. *Folia Primatologica, 46*, 118-124.

Gitlan, M. J., & Pasnau, R. O. (1989). Psychiatric syndromes linked to reproductive function in women: A review of current knowledge. *American Journal of Psychiatry, 146*, 1413-1422.

Giovannini, M. J. (1992). The relevance of gender in postpartum emotional disorders. In B. V. Reid, & T. L. Whitehead (Eds.), *Gender Constructs and Social Issues* (pp. 209-229). Urbana: University of Illinois Press.

Glinoer, D., de Nayer, P., Bourdoux, P., Lemone, M., Robyn, C., van Steirtegham, A., Kinthaert, J., & Lejeune, B. (1990). *Journal of Clinical Endocrinology and Metabolism, 71*, 276-287.

Goodlin, B. L., & Sackett, G. P. (1983). Parturition in Macaca nemestrina. *American Journal of Primatology, 4*, 283-307.

Gotlib, I. H., Whiffen, V. E., Mount, J. H., Milne, K., & Cordy, N. I. (1989). Prevalence rates and demographic characteristics associated with depression in pregnancy and the postpartum. *Journal of Consulting and Clinical Psychology, 57*, 269-274.

Gotlib, I. H., Whiffen, V. E., Wallace, P. M., & Mount, J. H. (1991). Prospective investigation of postpartum depression: Factors involved in onset and recovery. *Journal of Abnormal Psychology, 100*, 122-132.

Grazioli, R. & Terry, D. (2000). The role of cognitive vulnerability and stress in the prediction of postpartum depressive symptomatology. *British Journal of Clinical Psychology, 39*, 329-347.

Hackel, L.S., & Ruble, D. N. (1992). Changes in the marital relationship after the first baby is born: Predicting the impact of expectancy discrimination. *Journal of Personality and Social Psychology, 62*, 944-957.

Halpern, L., Anders, T., & Garcia Coll, C. (1994). Infant temperament: Is there a relation to sleep-wake states and maternal nighttime behavior? *Infant Behavior & Development, 17*, 255-263.

Handley, S. L., Dunn, T. L., Waldron, G., & Baker, J. M. (1980). Tryptophan, cortisol and puerperal mood. *British Journal of Psychiatry, 136*, 498-508.

Hapgood, C. C., Elkind, G. S., & Wright, J.J. (1988). Maternity blues: Phenomena and relationship to later postpartum depression. *Australian New Zealand Journal of Psychiatry, 22*, 299-306.

Harlow, H. F., Harlow, M. K., & Hansen, E. W. (1963). The maternal affectional system of rhesus monkeys. In H. Rheingold (Ed.), *Maternal behavior in mammals* (pp. 254-281). New York: Wiley.

Harris, B. (1980). Prospective trial of L-tryptophan in maternity blues. *British Journal of Psychiatry, 137*, 233-235.

Harris, B., Lovett, L., Newcombe, R. G., Read, G. F., & Walker, R. (1994). Maternity blues and major endocrine changes: Cardiff puerperal mood and hormone study II. *British Medical Journal, 308*, 949-954.

Harris, B., Parkes, A. B., & Phillips, D. I. H. (1992). Association between postpartum thyroid dysfunction and thyroid antibodies and depression. *British Medical Journal, 305*, 152.

Hatton, G. I., & Tweedle, C. D. (1982). Magnocellular neuropeptidergic neurons in hypothalamus: Increases in membrane apposition and number of specialized synapses from pregnancy to lactation. *Brain Research Bulletin, 8*, 197-204.

Hayes, M. J., Roberts, S. M., & Stowe, R. (1996). Early childhood co-sleeping: Parent-child and parent-infant night-time interactions. *Infant Mental Health Journal, 17*, 348-357.

Hayworth, J., Little, B. C., Bonham Carter, S., Raptopolus, P., Priest, Z. G., & Sandler, M. A. (1980). A predictive study of postpartum depression: Some predisposing characteristics. *British Journal of Medical Psychology, 53*, 161-167.

Herzog, A., & Deitre, T. (1976). Psychotic reactions associated with childbirth. *Diseases of the Nervous System, 37*, 229-235.

Hewlett, S. A (1986). *A lesser life: The myth of women's liberation in America*. New York: Warner.

Hobfoll, S. E., Ritter, C, Lavin, J., & Hulsizer, M. R. (1995). Depression prevalence and incidence among inner-city pregnant and postpartum women. *Journal of Consulting and Clinical Psychology, 63(3)*, 445-453.

Hock, E., & DeMeis, D. K. (1990). Depression in mothers of infants: The role of maternal employment. *Developmental Psychology, 26*, 285-292.

Hopkins, J. (1984). Postpartum depression: A critical review. *Psychological Bulletin, 95*, 498-515.

Hopkins, J., Campbell, S. B., & Marcus, M. (1987). Role of infant-related stressors in postpartum depression. *Journal of Abnormal Psychology, 96(3)*, 237-241.

Ieni, J. R., & Thurmond, J. B. (1985). Maternal aggression in mice: Effects of treatments with PCPA, 5-HT receptor antagonists. *European Journal of Pharmacology, 111*, 211-220.

Inwood, D. G. (Ed.). (1985). *Recent advances in postpartum depression*. Washington, DC: American Psychiatric Press.

Jolivet, A., Blanchier, H., Gautray, J. P., & Dhem, N. (1974). Blood cortisol variations during late pregnancy and labor. *American Journal of Obstetrics and Gynecology, 119*, 775-783.

Jordan, B. (1980). *Birth in Four Cultures*. Montreal: Eden Press.

Kendell, R. E., Chalmers, J. C., & Platz, C. (1987). Epidemiology of puerperal psychoses. *British Journal of Psychiatry, 150*, 662-673.

Kendell, R. E., McGuire, R. J., & Connor, Y. (1981). Mood changes in the first three weeks following childbirth. *Journal of Affective Disorders, 3*, 317-326.

Kendell, R., Rennie, D., Clarke, J., & Dean, C. (1981). The social and obstetric correlates of psychiatric admissions in the puerperium. *Psychological Medicine, 11*, 341-350.

Keverne, E. B. (1988). Central mechanisms underlying the neural and neuroendocrine determinants of maternal behavior. *Psychoneuroendocrinology, 13*, 127-141.

Keverne, E. B., Levy, F., Poindrom, P., & Lindsay, D. R. (1983). Vaginal stimulation: An important determinant of maternal bonding in sheep. *Science, 219*, 81-83.

Kinsley, C. H., & Bridges, R. S. (1986). Opiate involvement in postpartum aggression in rats. *Pharmacology, Biochemistry, and Behavior, 25*, 1007-1011.

Klaus, M. H. & Kennel, J. H. (1970). Human maternal behavior at first contact with her young. *Pediatrics, 46*, 187-192.

Krasnegor, N. A., & Bridges, R. S. (1990). *Mammalian Parenting*. New York: Oxford University Press.

Kumar, R., Brown, N., Campbell, I.C., Davies, A., Marks, M. N., McIvor, R.J., Papdopoulos, A., Wieck, A. & Checkley, S.A. (1994). Neuroendocrine and psychosocial correlates of psychotic and non-psychotic postpartum mental illnesses. *Neuropsychpharmacology, 10*, 903S.

Kumar, R. & Robson, K. (1984). A prospective study of emotional disorders in childbearing women. *British Journal of Psychiatry, 144*, 35-47.

Lee, S. R. (1982). Postpartum emotional disorders. *American Family Physician, 26*, 197-201.

LeVine, R.A. (1977). Child rearing as cultural adaptation. In H. Leiderma, S. Tulkin & A. Rosenfeld (Eds.). *Culture and Infancy*. New York: Academic Press.

Logsdon, M.C., McBride, A.B. & Birkimer, J.C. (1994). Social support and postpartum depression. *Research in Nursing & Health, 17*, 449-457.

Logsdon, M. & Usui, W. (2001). Psychosocial predictors of postpartum depression in diverse groups of women. *Western Journal of Nursing Research, 23(6)*, 563-574.

Lowry, P.J. (1993) Corticotropin-releasing factor and its binding protein in human plasma. *Ciba Foundation Symposium, 172*, 108-115.

Marks, M. N., Wieck, A., Checkley, S. A., & Kumar R. (1991). Life stress and post-partum psychosis: a preliminary report. *British Journal of Psychiatry, 10*, 45-49.

Martinez-Schallmoser, L., Telleen, S., & MacMullen, N. J. (2003). The effect of social support and acculturation on postpartum depression in Mexican American women. *Journal of Transcultural Nursing, 14*, 329-338.

McGorry, P., & Connell, S. (1990). The nosology and prognosis of puerperal psychosis: A review. *Comprehensive Psychiatry, 32(6)*, 519-534.

McIvor, R. J., Davies, R. A., Wieck, A., Marks, M. N., Brown, N., Campbell, I. C., Checkley, S. A., & Kumar, R. (1996). he growth hormone response to apomorphine at 4 days postpartum in women with a history of major depression. *Journal of Affective Disorders, 40*, 131-136.

McKenna, J. J., Thoman, E. B., Anders, T. F., Sadeh, A., Schecchtman, V. L., & Glotzbach, S. F. (1993). Infant-parent co-sleeping in an evolutionary perspective: Implications for understanding infant sleep development and the Sudden Infant Death Syndrome. *Sleep, 16*, 263-282.

McLean, M., Thompson, D., Zhang, H. P., Brinsmead, M., & Smith, R. (1994). Corticotrophin-releasing hormone and beta-endorphin in labor. *European Journal of Endocrinology, 13*, 167-172.

Misri, S, Kostaras, X., Fox, D., & Kostaras, D. (2000) The impact of partner support in the treatment of postpartum depression. *Canadian Journal of Psychiatry, 45*, 554-58.

Moltz, H. J., & Kilpatrick, S. J. (1980). Pheromonal control of maternal behavior. In R. W. Bell & W. P. Smotherman (Eds.), *Maternal influences and early behavior* (pp. 135-154). New York: Plenum Press.

Montagu, A. (1981). After office hours: Pseudocyesis, a review. *Obstetrics and Gynecology, 51*, 627-631.

Morelli, G. A., Rogoff, B., & Oppenheim, D. (1992). Cultural variation in infants' sleeping arrangement: Questions of independence. *Developmental Psychology, 28*, 604-610.

Muret-Wagstaff, S., & Moore, S.G. (1989). The Hmong in America: Infant behavior and rearing practices. In Nugent, J. K., Lester, B.M. & Brazelton, T.B. (Eds.). *The Cultural Context of Infancy*. (pp.319-339). Norwood, N.J.: Ablex Publishing.

Nahas, V. & Amasheh, N. (1999) Culture care meanings and experiences of postpartum depression among Jordanian Australian women: A transactional study. *Journal of Transcultural Nursing, 10*, 37-45.

Neter, E., Collins, N. L., Lobel, M., & Dunkel-Schetter, C. (1995). Psychosocial predictors of postpartum depressed mood in socioeconomically disadvantaged women. Women's Health: *Research on Gender, Behavior & Policy, 1*, 51-75.

Nott, P. N. (1987). Extent, timing and persistence of emotional disorders following childbirth. *British Journal of Psychiatry, 151*, 523-527.

Nott, P. N., Franklin, M., Armitage, C., & Gelder, M. G. (1976). Hormonal changes and mood in the puerperium. *British Journal of Psychiatry, 128*, 379-383.

Numan, M., Rosenblatt, J. S., Komisaruk, B. R. (1977). Medial preoptic area and onset of maternal behavior in the rat. *Journal of Comparative and Physiological Psychology, 91*, 146-164.

Numan, M., & Numan, M. (1996). A lesion and neuranatomical tract-tracing analysis of the role of the bed nucleus of the stria terminalis in retrieval behavior and other aspects of maternal responsiveness in rats. *Developmental Psychobiology, 29*, 23-51.

Oakley, A. (1980). *Women Confined: Towards a Sociology of Childbirth*. Oxford: Martin Robertson.

O'Hara, M. (1986). Social support, life events, and depression during pregnancy and the puerperium. *Archives of General Psychiatry, 43*, 569-573.

O'Hara, M. W., Neunaber, D. J., & Zekoski, E. M. (1984). Prospective study of postpartum depression: Prevalence, course, and predictive factors. *Journal of Abnormal Psychology, 93(2)*, 158-171.

O'Hara, M. W., Rehm, L. P., & Campbell, S. B. (1982). Predicting depressive symptomology: Cognitive-behavioral models and postpartum depression. *Journal of Abnormal Psychology, 91*, 457-461.

O'Hara, M. W., Rehm, L. P., & Campbell, S. B. (1983). Postpartum depression: A role for social network and life stress variables. *Journal of Nervous and Mental Disease, 171*, 336-341.

O'Hara, M. W., Schlechte, J. A., Lewis, D. A., & Varner, M. W. (1991). Controlled prospective study of postpartum mood disorders: Psychological, environmental, and hormonal variables. *Journal of Abnormal Psychology, 100*, 63-73.

O'Hara, M. W., Zekowski, E. M., Phillips, L. H., & Wright, E. J. (1990). Controlled prospective study of postpartum mood disorders: Comparison of childbearing and nonchildbearing women. *Journal of Abnormal Psychology, 99*, 3-15.

Ostermeyer, M. C. (1983). Maternal aggression. In R. W. Elwood (Ed.), *Parental behavior of rodents* (pp. 151-179). Chichester: Wiley.

Owens, N. W. (1975). Social play behavior in free-living baboons, Papio anubils. *Animal Behavior, 23*, 387-408.

Paul, S. M., & Purdy, R. H. (1992). Neuroactive steroids. *Official Publication of the Federation of American Societies for Experimental Biology, 6*, 2311-2322.

Paykel, E., Emms, E., Fletcher, J., & Rassaby, E. (1980). Life events and social support in puerperal depression. *British Journal of Psychiatry, 136*, 339-346.

Pecins-Thompson, M., & Bethea, C. L. (1999). Ovarian steroid regulation of serotonin-1A autoreceptor messenger RNA expression in the dorsal raphe of rhesus macaques. *Neuroscience, 89*, 267-277.

Pederson, C. A., & Prange, Jr., A. J. (1979). Induction of maternal behavior in virgin rats after intracerebroventricular administration of oxytocin. *Proceedings of the National Academy of Sciences USA, 76*, 6661-6665.

Perlmutter, L. S., Tweedle, C. D., & Hatton, G. I. (1984). Neuronal-glial plasticity in the supraoptic dendritic zone: Dedritic bundling and double synapse formation at parturition. *Neuroscience, 13*, 769-779.

Pfost, K. S., Stevens, M. J., & Lum, C. U. (1990). The relationship of demographic variables, antepartum depression, and stress to postpartum depression. *Journal of Clinical Psychology, 46(5)*, 588-592.

Pitt, B. (1969). "Atypical" depression following childbirth. *British Journal of Psychiatry, 114*, 1325-1335.

Pop, V.J., de Rooy, H. A., Vader, H.L., van der Heide, D., van Son, M., Komproe, I. H., Essed, G. G., & de Geus, C.A. (1991). Postpartum thyroid dysfunction and depression in an unselected population. *New England Journal of Medicine, 325(5)*, 371

Rehman, A.U., St. Clair, D. & Platz, C. (1990) Puerperal insanity in the 19th and 20th centuries. *British Journal of Psychiatry, 156*, 861-865.

Richman, J. A., Raskin, V. D., & Gaines, C. (1991). Gender roles, social support, and postpartum depressive symptomatology. *The Journal of Nervous and Mental Disease, 179(3)*, 139-147.

Rosenblatt, J. S. (1965). The basis of synchrony in the behavioral interaction between the mother and her offspring in the laboratory rat. In B. M. Foss (Ed.), *Determinants of infant behavior* (Vol. 3, pp. 3-41). London: Methuen.

Rothbart, M. K., Derryberry, D., & Posner, M. I. (1994). A psychobiological approach to the development of temperament. In J. E. Bates & T. D. Wachs (Eds.), *Temperament:*

Individual differences at the interface of biology and behavior (pp. 83-116). Washington, D.C.: American Psychological Association.

Russell, J., Douglas, A., & Ingram, C. (2001). Brain preparations for maternity – adaptive changes in behavioral and neuroendocrine systems during pregnancy and lactation. An overview. In J.A. Russell, A.J. Douglas, R.J. Windle, C.D. Ingram (Eds.), *Progress in Brain Research*, Vol. 133 (pp. 3-38). Amsterdam: Elsevier Science B.V.

Rutter, M. (1991). A fresh look at "maternal deprivation." In P. Bateson (Ed.), *The development and integration of behavior* (pp. 331-374). Cambridge: Cambridge University Press.

Sandman, C. A., Wadha, P. D., Chica-Demet, A., Dunkel-Schetter, C., & Porto, M. (1997). Maternal stress, HPA activity, and fetal/infant outcome. *Annals of the New York Academy of Sciences, 814*, 266-175.

Saucier, J. F., Bernazzani, O., Bogeat, F. (1995). La contribution de variables sociales á la prédiction de la depression postnatale. *Santé Mentale au Québec, 20*, 35-58.

Seguin, L., Potvin, L., St. Denis, M., & Loisell, J. (1999). Depressive symptoms in the late postpartum among low socioeconomic status women. *Birth, 26*, 157-163.

Shoeb, I. H., & Hassan, G. A. (1990). Postpartum psychosis in the Assir Region of Saudi Arabia. *British Journal of Psychiatry, 157*, 427-430.

Siegel, H. I., & Rosenblatt, J. S. (1975). Hormonal basis of hysterectomy-induced maternal behavior during pregnancy in the rat. *Hormones and Behavior, 6*, 211-222.

Steklis, H. D., & Kling, A. (1985). Neurobiology of affiliative behavior in nonhuman primates. In M. Reite & T. Field (Eds.), *The psychobiology of attachment and separation* (pp. 93-134). Orlando, FL: Academic Press.

Stern, J. M., Goldman, L., Levine, S. (1973). Pituitary-adrenal responsiveness during lactation in rats. *Neuroendocrinology, 12*, 179-191.

Stern & Kruckman. (1983) Multi-disciplinary perspectives on post-partum depression: an anthropological critique. *Social Science and Medicine, 17*, 1027-1041.

Stuchbery, M., Matthey, S., & Barnett, B. (1998) Postnatal depression and social supports in Vietnamese, Arabic, and Anglo-Celtic mothers. *Soc Psychiatry Psychiatr Epidemiol, 33*, 483-490.

Super, C., & Harkness, S. (1982). The infants niche in rural Kenya and metropolitan Kenya. In L. L. Adler (Ed.) Cross-cultural research at issue (pp. 47-55). New York: Academic Press.

Susman, V. L., & Katz, J. L. (1988). Weaning and depression: another postpartum complication. *American Journal of Psychiatry, 145*, 498-501.

Svare, B. (1981). Infanticide: Genetic, developmental and hormonal influences in mice. *Physiology and Behavior, 27*, 921-927.

Thomas, A., & Chess, S. (1977). Temperament and development. New York: Brunner Mazel.

Tod, E. D. M. (1964). Puerperal depression, a prospective epidemiological study. *Lancet, 2*, 1264-1266.

Trivers, R. L. (1972). Parental investment and sexual selection. In B. Campbell (Ed.), *Sex selection and the descent of man* 1871-1971 (pp. 136-179). Chicago: Aldine.

Tronick, E.Z., Winn, S., & Morelli, G.A. (1985). Multiple caretaking in the context of human evolution: Why don't the Efe know the Western prescription for child care. In M. Reite & T. Field (Eds.) *Psychobiology of attachment*. New York: Academic Press, pp. 293-322.

Troy, N.W. (1995). The time of first holding of the infant and maternal self-esteem related to feelings of maternal attachment. *Women & Health, 22*, 59-72.

Videbeck, & Gouliaev (1995). First admission with puerperal psychosis: 7-14 years of follow-up. *Acta Psychiatrica Scandinavica, 91*, 167-173.

Wadwa, P.D., Porto, M., Garite, T. J., Chicz-DeMet, A. & Sandman, C. A. (1998). Maternal CRH level in the early third trimester predict length of gestation in human pregnancy. *American Journal of Obstetrics and Gynecology, 179*, 1079-1085.

Walfish, P. G., Meyerson, J., Provias, J. P., Vargas, M. T., & Papsin, F. R. (1992). Prevalence and characteristics of post-partum thyroid dysfunction: Results of a survey from Toronto, Canada. *Journal of Endocrinological Investigation, 15*, 265-272.

Walsh, C. J., Fleming, A. S., Lee, A., & Magnusson, J. E. (1996). The effects of olfactory and somatosensory desensitization on Fos-like immunoreactivity in the brains of pup-exposed postpartum rats. *Behavioral Neuroscience, 110*, 134-153.

Warren , M. P., & Shortle, B. (1990). Endocrine correlates of human parenting: A clinical perspective. In K. Bridges (Ed.), *Endocrine Correlates of Human Parenting: A Clinical Perspective* (pp. 209-226). New York: Oxford.

Watson, J. P., Elliot, S. A., Rugg, A. J., & Brough, D. (1984). Psychiatric disorder in pregnancy and the first postnatal year. *British Journal of Psychiatry, 144*, 453-462.

Whiffen, V. E. (1988). Vulnerability to postpartum depression: A prospective multivariate study. *Journal of Abnormal Psychology, 97*, 467-474.

Whiffin, V. E. (1991). The comparison of postpartum with non-postpartum depression: a rose by any other name. *Journal of Psychiatry and Neuroscience, 16*, 160-165.

Whiffen, V. E. (1992). Is postpartum depression a distinct diagnosis? *Clinical Psychology Review, 12*, 485-508.

Whiffen, V. E., & Gotlib, I. H. (1993). Comparison of postpartum and nonpostpartum depression: Clinical presentation, psychiatric history, and psychosocial functioning. *Journal of Consulting and Clinical Psychology, 61*, 485-494.

Wieck, A., Kumar, R., Hirst, A. D., Marks, M. N., Checkley, S. A., & Campbell, I. C. (1991). Increased sensitivity of dopamine receptors and recurrence of affective psychosis after childbirth. *British Medical Journal, 303*, 613-617.

Wolke, D. & St. James-Roberts, I. (1987). Multi-method measurement of the early parent-infant system with easy and difficult newborns. In Rauh, H., Steinhausen, H.C. (Eds.), *Psychobiology and Early Development* (pp. 49-70). Amsterdam: North-Holland/Elsevier.

Yalom, I. P., Lunde, D. T., Moss, R. H., & Hamburg, D. A. (1968). Postpartum blues syndrome: A description and related variables. *Archives of General Psychiatry, 18*, 16-27.

Chapter II

POSTPARTUM DEPRESSION: LATIN-AMERICAN PERSPECTIVES

Johann Vega-Dienstmaier[1], and Maria I. Zapata-Vega[2]*
[1]Universidad Peruana Cayetano Heredia, Lima, Peru;
[2]Mount Sinai School of Medicine, New York, USA

ABSTRACT

In the past two decades there has been increasing recognition that mood disorders, particularly depression, are a significant cause of pregnancy-related morbidity. Latin-American researchers have been actively contributing to the field of perinatal psychiatry. This article presents a review of the scientific literature on postpartum depression, available in MEDLINE and LILACS/BIREME databases, developed in Latin-American countries including studies conducted mostly in Brazil, Peru, and Chile. Furthermore, due to the known vast migration of Latin-American individuals into developed countries, selected studies on postpartum depression in women of Latino heritage in the United States of America were also reviewed.

Significant efforts involving the adaptation and validation of widely used instruments for the assessment of postpartum depression in Spanish and Portuguese language, such as the Edinburgh Postnatal Depression Scale, have been reported.

Estimates of the prevalence of depression in puerperal women varied from 5.92% and 48% in different clinical settings. The time at which the maternal assessments were conducted ranged from as early as one day to after up to one year postpartum.

Demographic characteristics, availability of social and financial resources, affective support from partners and family, history of depression and/or other psychiatric symptomatology, other pregnancy-related pathologies, premature births, and neonatal illness, among others, have been consistently identified as associated risk factors for the development of postpartum depression in different studies throughout Latino-America.

---

* Correspondence concerning this article should be addressed to Dr. Johann Vega-Dienstmaier. Alfredo León 114 – 1004, Lima 18, Perú. E-mail: johannvega@yahoo.com

Similar findings, in addition to migration and acculturation factors, may play a roll in the development of depression in Latino women in the USA.

The impact of perinatal depression in the wellbeing of mothers and their children, and perinatal and pediatric care and beneficial interventions for risk groups such as premature children were addressed in other contributions.

The need for appropriate assessment, diagnosis, and treatment of postpartum depression, and the development of preventive strategies and specific services are discussed.

Keywords: Postpartum Depression, Latino-America, Latinos, Epidemiology, Risk Factors

INTRODUCTION

Since the times of Hippocrates (4th Century BC), it was known that there was some association between childbirth and mental disorders (Miller, 1999). In most recent times, there has been growing evidence that mood disorders, particularly depression, are a significant cause of pregnancy-related morbidity.

Disorders in the postpartum state may involve the recurrence of preexisting mental conditions or the onset of a new disorder; the severity may range from the most benign syndromes such as "postpartum blues" or "baby blues" to other potentially lethal conditions like postpartum psychosis (Wyszynski & Lusskin, 2005).

Research on postpartum disorders have been conducted mostly in industrialized countries and presented in the scientific literature in English language. Nevertheless, researchers in other geographical areas have made significant contributions to the field.

This article is intended to review the studies on postpartum depression (PPD) developed in Latino-America and published in the international medical literature. In addition, due to the growing number of women of Hispanic/Latino origin in developed countries like the USA (US Census, 2000), studies conducted on this particular population were also reviewed.

METHODOLOGY

The authors conducted a literature search in the LILACS/BIREME and Medline databases searching for all original articles published until March 2006. Inclusion criteria were as followed: only original papers with an abstract, conducted in any Latin-American country or involving Latino women in the USA, and addressing "postpartum", "postnatal", "perinatal", or "maternal" depression, as well as, early mother-child interactions.

The first search was conducted in LILACS using the keywords: "depression" and "postpartum" or "puerperium". A second search was conducted in Medline using the following keywords: "postpartum depression" and "Latinos/Hispanics", "Latino-America", "Spanish", "Portuguese", names of the eighteen Spanish-speaking Latin-American countries and "Brazil".

SEARCH RESULTS

The search through the LILACS/BIREME database yielded 22 original articles in Spanish or Portuguese language. The second search in Medline resulted in a total of 23 papers, meeting the above criteria and documenting studies on PPD conducted in Latin-American countries (n= 11, five of these articles were already included in the LILACS search results) or on Latino women in the USA (n= 12). Full articles were retrieved through the Latin-American and Caribbean Center on Health Sciences Information.

Articles were classified into four areas: validation of instruments for the assessment of PPD, epidemiology of the disorder, risk factors, and impact on mother-child interaction.

INSTRUMENTS FOR THE ASSESSMENT OF POSTPARTUM DEPRESSION

The DSM-IV-TR added the specifier "postpartum onset" to the diagnosis of Major Depressive Disorder, whenever the depressive episode occurs within 4 weeks after childbirth, it is not considered as a separate class of affective disorder. However, most studies do not use standardized criteria and more frequently diagnose the presence of depression based on positive scores using depression assessment instruments. In Latino-America significant efforts have been made to adapt and validate widely used instruments for, specifically, the assessment of postpartum depression in Spanish or Portuguese language.

Most studies involved the validation of the Spanish version of the Edinburgh Postnatal Depression Scale (EPDS), originally developed in England (Cox et al., 1987), specifically reported in Peru (Vega-Dienstmaier et al., 2002) and Chile (Jadresic et al., 1995; Alvarado et al., 1992b); and its Portuguese version studied in Brazil (Santos et al., 1999). A summary of the main psychometric findings for each study are showed in Table 1, and in addition, we calculated the number-needed-to-diagnose (NND) based on the sensitivity reported by the investigators for the best cut-off points (Bandolier, 1996).

Brazil

The Portuguese version of the EPDS was studied in the city of Brasilia (Santos et al., 1999), where a sample of 236 women, and a sub-sample of 69 subjects for additional statistical analysis, was assessed at 6-24 weeks after childbirth. The cut-off score found to have the lowest NND (1.52) was 10.5, with a sensitivity of 84% and specificity of 82%.

Chile

Two studies validating the EPDS were conducted in Chile by different research teams (Alvarado et al., 1992b; Jadresic et al., 1995). Both studies in this country suggests 9.5 as the best cut-off score for detection of depression, with a calculated NND of 1.51 (sensitivity= 85.71% and specificity=80.41%) in the first one and of 1.25 (sensitivity= 100% and specificity= 80%) in the second one.

Another scale, the Beck Depression Inventory (BDI), was also validated in Chile for its use in the screening of pregnancy and postpartum depression (Alvarado et al., 1993b). A cut-off point of 13.5 for this scale had the lowest calculated NND of all instruments reviewed here for the diagnosis of PPD (NND=1.21, sensitivity=85.71% and specificity= 96.91%). This finding does not support the idea that for the assessment of PPD, the use of specific instruments for puerperium like the EPDS is needed.

Table 1: Validation of assessment instruments for PPD: psychometric properties and best cut-off scores.

Country (City) Author/ Year	Scale	Language	Sample size	Time after child's birth	Cronbach's alpha	Diagnostic reference	Cut-off point	Sensibility	Specificity	NND
BRAZIL (Brasilia) Santos et al., 1999	EPDS	Portuguese	N=236 (and sub-sample of N= 69)	6-24 weeks	0.8	Major/minor depression- RDC	10.5	84	82	1.52
CHILE (Santiago) Jadresic et al., 1995	EPDS	Spanish	N=108 (11 depressed)	2-3 months	0.77	Major/minor depression RDC / PAS	9.5	100	80	1.25
CHILE (Santiago & Codegua) Alvarado et al., 1993b	BDI	Spanish	N=28, depressed; N=97, non-depressed	8 weeks	0.848	Depressive Episode- DSM-III-R	13.5	85.71	96.91	1.21
CHILE (Santiago & Codegua) Alvarado et al., 1992b	EPDS	Spanish	N=28, depressed; N=97, non-depressed	8 weeks	0.844	Depressive Episode- DSM-III-R	9.5 12.5	85.71 71.43	80.41 94.85	1.51 1.51
PERU (Lima) Vega-Dienstmaier et al., 2002	EPDS	Spanish	N=19, depressed; N=302, non-depressed	1st year	0.7043	Major Depression- SCID / DSM-IV	7.5 13.5	100 84.21	25.50 79.47	3.92 1.57
USA Beck & Gable, 2005	PDSS	Spanish	N=150	2-12 weeks	0.95	Major/minor depression- SCID / DSM-IV	60	84	84	1.47
	PDSS 7-Item				0.79		13	84	80	1.56
USA Beck & Gable, 2003	PDSS	Spanish	N=377	12 weeks	0.95	-	-	-	-	-

EPDS = Edinburgh Postnatal Depression Scale, PDSS = Postpartum Depression Screening Scale, BDI = Beck Depression Inventory, PAS = Psychiatric Assessment Schedule, RDC = Research Diagnostic Criteria, SCID = Structured Clinical Interview for DSM-IV.

NND = Number-needed-to-diagnose = {1 / [Sensitivity - (1 - Specificity)]}

Peru

The study of the EPDS in Peru, included women evaluated within the first year after childbirth and found, for a total score of 13.5, a sensitivity of 84.21% and a specificity of 79.47% (Vega-Dienstmaier et al., 2002). It also reported that the items assessing feelings of been anxious or worried, feelings of getting overwhelmed, frequency of crying spells, and feelings of been scared or panicky, contributed the most to the predictive ability of the instrument. These findings may suggest that anxiety is a predominant aspect in the evaluation of postpartum depression. A higher cut-off point in this study may be related to the fact that only women diagnosed with "major" depression were included as cases, whereas other validation studies included also subjects with "minor" depression.

Spanish-Speaking Women in the USA

In the USA, the Postpartum Depression Screening Scale (PDSS), the original 35-item version and a 7-item Short Form, were translated into Spanish (Beck et al., 2003) and its psychometric properties were found to be "slightly lower, but still in the acceptable range" when compared to the measurements of the original English version (Beck & Gable, 2003 and 2005).

EPIDEMIOLOGY OF POSTPARTUM DEPRESSION IN LATINO-AMERICA

International studies on postpartum depression estimate its prevalence between 10 and 15% (Beck 2001; O'Hara & Swain, 1996); however, studies around the world have shown a great heterogeneity of results. Symptoms, complaints, and syndromes may vary across cultures; therefore, cross-cultural considerations are to be taken when attempting to determine the epidemiology of this disorder (Halbreich & Karkun, 2006).

An additional challenge for clinicians and researchers seems the discrimination between the diagnosis of "postpartum depression" versus more benign and transient conditions such as "postpartum blues" or "postpartum dysphoria" presented in the very first days after childbirth.

Studies reporting prevalence of depressive symptoms in Latino-America and in Hispanic women in the USA are shown in Table 2. Prevalence estimates of depressive symptoms, in Latin-American countries, without making a distinction between "blues" and postpartum depression, ranged between 6.8% and 48%. Almost all reports described the use of the EPDS or other instruments for the diagnosis of depression, and the authors cited, in the majority of cases, previous adaptation and validation of the instrument in their targeted population. The assessment of depressive symptoms was, in most cases, conducted only once and in the early puerperium; therefore, symptoms may represent postpartum dysphoria or "blues". Study subjects were recruited not only in specialized obstetric settings, but also in primary care clinics and during pediatric visits.

Brazil

Eight studies conducted in Brazil and reporting data on postpartum depressive symptomatology were found. One of these studies used "postpartum blues" scales, but no reference to previous validation of these instruments in the population was cited. The prevalence of depression, as measured by the "blues" scales, varied within 30.1% - 32.7% by the 10th day (Faisal-Cury et al., 2004). Additionally, Rohde et al. (1997), used the Blues Questionnaire (Kennerley & Gath, 1989) to assessed postpartum women (n=86) on a daily basis during the first 8 days and compared them with a sample of 'out of postpartum' female hospital workers (n=75), finding that the symptomatic peak was reached at the 5th day, however no specific prevalence was reported.

The EPDS was used in three studies, using cut-off scores above 12 or 13 (Moreno et al., 2004; Coutinho et al., 2002; Da Silva et al., 1998). The study by Da Silva et al. (1998) assessed the subjects on six monthly home visits and found a rate of 42.8%, however, only a small sample (N=33) of puerperal women were enrolled. Larger studies using the EPDS found prevalence rates between 22.2 % and 32.9%, recruiting, in both cases, women bringing their children for pediatric visits. They, respectively, assessed 73 women at 3 to 6 months postpartum (Coutinho et al., 2002), and 123 women between 8 and 12 weeks after childbirth (Moreno et al., 2004).

Two other studies were conducted in the city of Pelotas. One study used the Hamilton Depression Scale (HAM-D) on 410 women interviewed 1-1.5 months after childbirth; it found occurrence of depression in 19.1% of cases (Moraes et al., 2006). The other study, evaluated the presence of depressive symptoms not only in the mother but also in the child's father (N = 386 couples) (Pinheiro et al., 2006). In this case, the BDI was used during home visits at 6 to 12 weeks after childbirth, and found a prevalence of 23.6% of maternal depression and 11.9% of paternal depression. The presence of paternal depression was higher among men whose wives had moderate or severe depression.

An additional report by Luis & Oliveira (1998) documented the review of 135 cases that met International Classification of Diseases-9th Edition (ICD-9) criteria for "Mental Disorders in Pregnancy, Childbirth, and Puerperium" evaluated in psychiatric emergency services and obstetrics clinic in the city of Ribeirão Preto. Results were not specified for each perinatal phase, but it was noteworthy that 8.1% of the cases with the above broad diagnosis presented with depressive symptoms, the majority related to suicide attempts. Since it seemed that these evaluations necessitated some level of emergency care, it could be anticipated that other serious disorders (e.g. psychosis) accounted for a considerable percentage of cases.

Chile

Five studies in Chile containing epidemiological data were identified. Clinical psychiatric interviews were conducted in two studies to appraise standardized diagnostic criteria. Evans et al. (2003) reported a 32.07% of depression in 106 women interviewed at 5 to 6 months after childbirth based on ICD-10 criteria. Other authors reported a prevalence of depression of 20.5 - 22.4% in 125 women interviewed at 2 to 8 weeks postpartum using DSM-III-R criteria (Alvarado et al., 1992a and 2000).

Hasbun et al. (1999) used two scales, HAM-D and EPDS, in 103 women assessed at the 3rd day postpartum and followed 43 of them to complete a second evaluation by the 12th week. At the 3rd day, the prevalence of depression ranged between 6.8% and 27.2%, and it increased by the 12th week to a range between 27.9% and 48%. The latter was the highest prevalence of PPD found in the studies reviewed for this report.

Two studies conducted by Jadresic and collaborators in 1995 and earlier in 1992, recruited women at 2 to 3 months postpartum. One study used the EPDS (n=542) and found a prevalence of 36.7% (Jadresic & Araya, 1995). Whereas, the earlier study, reported a prevalence of 10.2% using the *Cuestionario de Selección de Depressión* (CSD-20) by Florenzano et al. (1984) followed by a semi-structured psychiatric interview, using the Psychiatric Assessment Schedule (PAS), in addition to the EPDS on a smaller sample (n=108) (Jadresic et al., 1992a).

Costa Rica

Wolf et al. (2002) studied two samples of mothers of infants enrolled in a study on iron-deficiency anemia and infant behavior. Costa Rican mothers were interviewed about recollection of episodes of depressed mood following childbirth (at 12-23 months postpartum in one sample and after 5 years in the other); however this later interview did not distinguish between "baby blues" and more serious postpartum mood disorders. Dysphoric mood following delivery of a child was documented in 35% - 38% of the mothers included in these samples.

Peru

Postpartum "blues" were studied in 360 puerperal women in the city of Cuzco (Betalleluz & Quiroz, 1997). Women were assessed for "postpartum dysphoric syndrome" using items from the BDI and the Zung Self-Rating Anxiety Scale. The diagnosis was based on five established criteria: depressed mood, crying spells, sleep disturbance, anxiety, and mood changes / irritability / decreased attention span / forgetfulness. Women were recruited in the maternity wards of three local hospitals and interviewed at the first, fourth, and eight day after childbirth. It was found that 34.44% of the women developed the syndrome with a symptomatic peak at the third day.

Vega-Dienstmaier et al. (1999) studied a total of 425 women divided into 3 samples: nulliparous (n=41), up to one year postpartum (n=321), and over one year after childbirth (n=63). The assessment included the Structured Clinical Interview for DSM-IV (SCID) for current and past major depressive episodes, and other psychiatric disorders. The study found that 5.92% of women presented depressive symptoms in the first puerperal year, whereas in women whose children were over one year-old, the prevalence of major depression was 14.29%, this prevalence difference was statistically significant.

Table 2. Prevalence of postpartum depressive symptoms in Latin-American women and Hispanic women in the USA.

Country (City) Author, Year	Sample size	Evaluation setting	Time after child's birth	Scale (Cut-off point)	Prevalence of depressive symptoms
BRAZIL (Pelotas) Moraes et al., 2006	N=410	Home visits	30-45 days	HAM-D (Score≥18)	19.1%
BRAZIL (Pelotas) Pinheiro et al., 2006	N=386 couples	Home visits	6-12 weeks	BDI (Score≥10)	23.6% (Mothers) 11.9% (Fathers)
BRAZIL (Brasilia) Moreno et al., 2004	N=123	Pediatric clinic	8-12 weeks	EPDS (Score≥12)	22.2%
BRAZIL (São Paulo) Faisal-Cury et al., 2004	N=113	Obstetrics clinic	10th day	BDI (Score≥15)	15.9%
				Pitt's Blues Scale (Score > 20) or Stein's Blues Scale (Score >8)	30.1% and 32.7%
BRAZIL (Sao Paulo) Coutinho et al., 2002	N=73	Health Center, Pediatric visits	3-6 months	EPDS (Score≥13)	32.9%
BRAZIL (Rio de Janeiro) Da-Silva et al., 1998	N=33	Home visits	Monthly, for 6 months	EPDS (Score≥13)	42.8%
BRAZIL (Ribeirão Preto) Luis & Oliveira, 1998	N=135	Psychiatric Emergency & Obstetrics clinic (Chart review)	Not specified	ICD-9 Criteria for "Mental Disorders in Pregnancy, Childbirth and Puerperium" (648.4)	8.1%, of all cases reviewed. Not specified for postpartum period.
BRAZIL (Porto Alegre) Rohde et al., 1997	N=86, postpartum; N=75, controls	Maternity ward & home visits	Daily, for 8 days	Blues Questionnaire	Symptoms peak at 5th day. Specific prevalence not reported.
CHILE (Antofagasta) Evans et al., 2003	N=106	Obstetrics clinic	5-6 months	ICD-10 criteria (5 or more, for at least 2 weeks)	32.07%
CHILE Alvarado et al., 1992a & 2000	N=125	Three Primary Care Centers	2nd and 8th weeks	Psychiatric interview (based on DSM-III-R criteria)	20.5-22.4%
CHILE (Santiago) Hasbun et al., 1999	N=103	Two hospitals	3rd day (n= 103) and 12th week (n=43)	HAM-D (Score>10)	6.8% (3rd day) 27.9% (12th week)
				EPDS (Score≥10)	27.2% (3rd day) 48% (12th week)
CHILE (Santiago) Jadresic & Araya, 1995	N=542	Five Health Centers, Pediatric visits & Home visits	2-3 months	EPDS (Score≥10)	36.7%
CHILE (Santiago) Jadresic et al., 1992a	N=108	University diagnostic center, Home visits, & Pediatric visits	2-3 months	Major / minor depression CSD-20 PAS EPDS	10.2%
COSTA RICA (Hatillo & Desamparados) Wolf et al., 2002	N=151 (Hatillo) N=80 (Desamparados)	Home visits, Pediatric visits	5 years 12-23 months *	Episodes of "dysphoric mood" after childbirth	38.0% 35.0%

Table 2. (Continued)

Country (City) Author, Year	Sample size	Evaluation setting	Time after child's birth	Scale (Cut-off point)	Prevalence of depressive symptoms
PERU (Lima) Vega-Dienstmaier et al., 1999	N=384, postpartum; N=41, nulliparous	Family Planning & Pediatric Services	Within 1st year (n=321) and after 1 year (n=63)	Major depression SCID / DSM-IV	5.92% (1st year) and 14.29% (after 1 year)
PERU (Cuzco) Betalleluz et al., 1997	N=360	Obstetrics clinic	1st, 4th, and 8th day	"Postpartum dysphoric syndrome" based on items of BDI & ZSAS	34.44%
USA (San Mateo County) Chaudron et al., 2005	N=218	Telephone surveys (outreach program)	6-18 months	EPDS (Score≥10)	23%
USA (Tucson) Freeman et al., 2005	N=96 (53.2% of Hispanic ethnicity)	Pediatric visits	30-103 days	EPDS (Score≥12)	14.6% of he total sample (no specific data for Hispanic women was reported)

* Unclear information.
HAM-D = Hamilton Scale for Depression, BDI = Beck Depression Inventory, EPDS = Edinburgh Postnatal Depression Scale, CSD-20 = *Cuestionario de Selección de Depresión,* SCID = Structured Clinical Interview for DSM-IV, PAS = Psychiatric Assessment Schedule, CES-D = Center for Epidemiologic Studies - Depression scale, DIS = Diagnostic Interview Schedule, ZSAS = Zung Self-Rating Anxiety Scale.

Hispanic Women in the USA

Two recent studies on Hispanic women in the USA were found, both using the EPDS. One study by Chaudron et al. (2005) in San Mateo County, California, involved 218 women participants of a countywide initiative to improve comprehensive outreach services to pregnant women and those with children aged 4 and under. Women with children ages 6 - 18 months, most of them immigrants, were included and data was collected through telephone surveys using the EPDS. Twenty three percent of women scored positively to the EPDS. The other study (Freeman et al., 2005), conducted in Tucson, Arizona, does not present specific data on Latinas, but was considered in this review because the sample of 96 women was composed of over 50% of Hispanics. In this study, 14.6% of the total sample scored positively to the EPDS.

RISK FACTORS ASSOCIATED TO POSTPARTUM DEPRESSION

Risks factors found in association to PPD in Latin-American studies are shown in Table 3. The variables described here include: life events (stressors), socioeconomic status, demographic characteristics (e.g. age, ethnicity), educational level, social and family support, relationship with partner, expectations about the pregnancy, number of previous pregnancies, mental and general medical problems.

One of the most significant factors is the number of life events or stressors the mother needs to cope with. Life events had a strong association to PPD ($p<0.001$) in two studies conducted in Chile (Alvarado et al., 1994; Jadresic et al., 1992b). Among those stressors, the most relevant are the ones related to some risk to the pregnancy or the newborn, for example, low-weight at birth (Jadresic et al., 1992b), premature birth or some risk to the newborn's life (Eizirik, 1984). Other significant stressors include having an abortion immediately before the current pregnancy (Alvarado et al., 1994), having a close person with a serious illness or the onset of severe economic difficulties (Jadresic et al., 1992b).

A lower socio-economic status was associated to the development of PPD in Brazil (Moraes et al., 2006) and worries about pregnancy-related expenses were linked to postpartum dysphoria in Peru (Betalleluz & Quiroz, 1997). Similar findings in the work by Betalleluz & Quiroz (1997) in Peru and by Moraes et al. (2006) in Brazil documented a low number of prenatal visits as a factor associated to the development of depression in the puerperium.

Several studies reported that low educational level is a risk factor for the development of PPD (Moraes et al., 2006; Faisal-Curry et al., 2002; Vega-Dienstmaier et al., 1999; Howell et al., 2005). However, a study in Costa Rica found an association between "postpartum dysphoria" and higher level of education (Wolf et al., 2001). This finding may be explained by the fact that women were asked to remember the presence of postnatal dysphoria up to 5 years after childbirth; therefore, higher levels of education may have influenced the recollection of better-detailed information.

Inadequate social support has been identified also as a factor in some studies (Coutinho et al., 2002; Martinez-Schallmoser et al., 2003; Howell et al., 2005). Being away from her family or close friends or having serious conflicts with her own mother seems to be also linked to the development of PPD (Jadresic et al., 1992b). Other identified factors are those pertaining to the mother's relationship with her partner, among these: unsatisfactory relation with the partner before or after childbirth (Alvarado et al., 1992a), marital conflicts (Jadresic et al., 1992b), relational difficulties with the child's father (Moraes et al., 2006), limited presence or absence of the partner (Hasbun et al., 1999; Betalleluz & Quiroz, 1997), and been single, separated or widow (Moraes et al., 2006; Hasbun et al., 1999; Jadresic & Arraya, 1995).

Other factors found associated to PPD involved the mother's attitude and expectations attached to her pregnancy. For example: having contemplated to terminate the pregnancy or having in fact attempted to do it (Moraes et al., 2006), having a negative attitude towards the pregnancy (Alvarado et al., 1992a), and if the pregnancy was unplanned (Hasbun et al., 1999). Moraes et al. (2006) found a peculiar relationship between the preference for a child of male gender and the development of depression.

Having a larger number of children or previous pregnancies was found associated to PPD in several studies (Faisal-Curry et al., 2002; Hasbun et al., 1999; Vega-Dienstmaier et al., 1999). On the contrary, Da-Silva et al. (1998) found an opposite relation between the number of children and the risk for PPD.

Table 3. Risk Factors for the development of Postpartum Depression.

Country Author, Year	Criteria/scale to diagnose Postpartum Depression	Variables associated to Postpartum Depression	Significance of the association
Brazil Moraes et al., 2006	HAM-D (Score ≥ 18)	Low family income	P=0.005
		Low social class	P=0.025
		Poor maternal education	P=0.003
		Young maternal age	P=0.005
		Marital status: Single, separated or widow	P=0.012
		Poor prenatal care (low number of visits)	P=0.016
		Lack of support from child's father	P=0.030
		Thought of terminating pregnancy	P=0.005
		Tried to terminate pregnancy	P=0.031
		Preference for a child of male gender	P<0.001
Brazil Pinheiro et al., 2006	BDI	Paternal depression	P<0.001
Brazil Faisal-Curry et al., 2002	BDI (Score >15)	Lower educational level	P=0.004
		Having 3 or more children	P=0.004
		Not been a primiparous	P=0.008
		Having previous pregnancies	P=0.015
		6 or more years of marital life	P=0.036
		Ethnicity (White)	P=0.02
Brazil Da-Silva et al., 1998	EPDS (Score ≥ 13)	Ethnicity (Black)	P<0.05
		Fewer previous pregnancies	P<0.05
Brazil Eizirik, 1984	6 cards of the TAT by Welch et al. (1961)	Premature child	P<0.05
		Newborn with some life risk	P<0.05
Brazil Coutinho et al., 2002	EPDS	Dysphoria during current or after previous pregnancies	P=0.033
		Mother had a diagnosis of depression in her lifetime	P=0.005
		Poor social support from mother's family	P<0.05
Chile Evans et al., 2003	ICD-10	Some illness during pregnancy	Statist. Sig.*
		Child hospitalized as a newborn or while breast-fed	Statist. Sig.*
		History of previous depression	Statist. Sig.*
Chile Hasbun et al., 1999	EPDS HAM-D	Unexpected pregnancy	P=0.0041
		Having 3 or more children	P=0.034
		Absence of the child's father	P=0.003
		Vaginal delivery	P=0.009
		Conflicts with the child's father	P=0.0068
		Being a single mother	P=0.023
Chile Jadresic & Araya, 1995	EPDS	Familiar income (low)	P<0.01
		Single / widow (vs. married / living together)	P=0.01
Chile Alvarado et al., 1994	DSM-III-R	Having an abortion immediately before the pregnancy	P=0.048
		Life events	P<0.001
Chile Alvarado et al., 1993a	DSM-III-R	Urinary tract infection during pregnancy	P=0.039
		Stopping breast-feeding	P=0.015
Chile Alvarado et al., 1992a	DSM-III-R	Age extremes (< 19 or > 34 year-old)	P=0.021
		Depression during 3rd trimester	P<0.001
		Negative attitude towards pregnancy	P=0.011
		Unsatisfactory relation with partner before childbirth	P=0.018
		Unsatisfactory relation with partner after childbirth	P<0.001

Table 3. Risk Factors for the development of Postpartum Depression. (Continued)

Country Author, Year	Criteria/scale to diagnose Postpartum Depression	Variables associated to Postpartum Depression	Significance of the association
Chile Jadresic et al., 1992b	RDC	Life events in general	P<0.001
		Child with low-weight or small-size at birth	P<0.001
		Previously seen by a specialist due to emotional problems	P<0.01
		Being separated from family or close friend	P<0.01
		Severe economic problems	P<0.01
		Marital conflict	P<0.025
		Difficulties with breast-feeding	P<0.025
		Anxiety or depressive symptoms during pregnancy	P<0.025
		Development of varicose veins	P<0.025
		Having serious conflicts with her own mother	P<0.05
		Close person became seriously ill	P<0.05
		Having several urinary tract infections	P<0.05
Costa Rica Wolf et al., 2001	"Postpartum dysphoria"	Higher educational level	P=0.04
		Less crowded household	P=0.02
Peru Vega-Dienstmaier et al., 1999	SCID for DSM-IV	Obsessive-Compulsive Disorder	P=0.0004
		Past Major Depressive Episode	P=0.002
		Premenstrual dysphoric disorder	P=0.007
		Maternity blues	P=0.016
		Age < 25 year-old	P=0.018
		Young maternal age	B=-0.13, SE=0.08
		Lower educational level	B=-0.23, SE=0.15
		Larger number of pregnancies	B=-0.32, SE=0.28
		Obsessive-Compulsive Disorder	P=0.0004
Peru Betalleluz & Quiroz, 1997	"Postpartum dysphoric syndrome"	Insufficient prenatal care	P=0.009
		Non-complex occupation	P<0.05
		Worries about financial expenses	P<0.05
		Partner's absence	P<0.05
		Limited presence of the partner at home	P<0.05
		Poor support from the partner	P<0.05
		Sleep deprivation	P<0.05
		Excessive work	P<0.05
		Need to meet multiple demands simultaneously	P<0.05
		Mother's upbringing was under adverse circumstances	P<0.05
USA, Hispanic women Howell et al., 2005	2-items from the Primary Care Evaluation of Mental Disorders Procedure	Age < 25 year-old	P<0.01
		Educational level ≤ high school	P<0.05
		Infant colic	P<0.01
		Poor social support	P<0.01
		Less access to their health care providers	P<0.05
		Less self-efficacy in managing the infant and household affairs	P<0.01
		Physical symptoms	P<0.01
		Physical function limitations	P<0.01
USA, Hispanic women Beck et al., 2005	PDSS SCID	Marital status (single)	Statist. Signif.*
		Number of days postpartum (more)	Statist. Signif.*
		Puerto Rican ethnicity	Statist. Signif.*
		Delivery by cesarean-section	Statist. Signif.*

Table 3. Risk Factors for the development of Postpartum Depression .(Continued)

Country Author, Year	Criteria/scale to diagnose Postpartum Depression	Variables associated to Postpartum Depression	Significance of the association
USA, > 50% Hispanic sample Freeman et al., 2005	EPDS	Smoking	P=0.0025
		Family history of mental health problems	P=0.0093
USA, Mexican-American women Heilemann et al., 2004	CES-D	Mastery (inverse correlation)	<0.001
		Satisfaction with life (inverse correlation)	<0.001
		Resilience subscale 1: personal competence (inverse correlation)	<0.008
		Resilience subscale 2: Acceptance of self & life (inverse correlation)	<0.001
		Importance of spiritual beliefs (inverse correlation)	0.02
USA, Mexican-American women Martinez-Schallmoser et al., 2003	CES-D	Prenatal depression	P=0.0001
		Postpartum family health (inverse correlation)	P=0.0001
		Postpartum support need	P=0.03
		Prenatal support need	P<0.05
		Prenatal support satisfaction (inverse correlation)	P<0.05
		Prenatal conflict network size	P<0.05
		Postnatal support satisfaction (inverse correlation)	P<0.05
		Postnatal conflict network size	P<0.05

HAM-D = Hamilton Scale for Depression, BDI = Beck Depression Inventory, EPDS = Edinburgh Postnatal Depression Scale, TAT = Thematic Apperception Test, RDC= Research Diagnostic Criteria, ICD-10 = International Classification of Diseases- 10th revision, SCID = Structured Clinical Interview for DSM-IV, PDSS = Postpartum Depression Screening Scale, CES-D = Center for Epidemiologic Studies – Depression scale.
* Reported by authors as "statistically significant"

About mental illness, the history of depression at anytime prior to the puerperium was consistently found associated to PPD in several studies (Vega-Dienstmaier et al., 1999; Coutinho et al., 2002; Evans et al., 2003), particularly if the depressive episode occurred during the pregnancy (Jadresic et al., 1992b; Alvarado et al., 1992a; Martinez-Schallmoser et al., 2003). Other mental health conditions found to be risk factors were: Obsessive-compulsive disorder, premenstrual dysphoric disorder and "maternity blues" (Vega-Dienstmaier et al., 1999); also, having previously consulted a mental health specialist for emotional problems (Jadresic et al., 1992b), and the history of dysphoria after a previous pregnancy or during the present one (Coutinho et al., 2002). Other interesting and very important finding by Pinheiro et al. (2006) involved the association of maternal depression and the occurrence of paternal depression after childbirth.

Factors related to maternal and the newborn's general health were also linked to PPD: any pathology during the pregnancy (Evans et al., 2003), presence of significant physical symptoms (Howell et al., 2005), physical limitations (Howell et al., 2005), urinary tract infections (Alvarado et al., 1993a; Jadresic et al., 1992b), development of varicose veins (Jadresic et al., 1992b), child required to be hospitalized as a newborn or while still being breast-fed (Evans et al., 2003), problems related to breast-feeding (Alvarado et al., 1993a; Jadresic et al., 1992b) and a child suffering from colics (Howell et al., 2005).

Young maternal age seems a consistent finding connected to PPD (Moraes et al., 2006; Vega-Dienstmaier et al., 1999; Howell et al., 2005; Alvarado et al., 1992a). Maternal age over 34 year-old was also found as a risk factor (Alvarado et al., 1992a).

Ethnicity represents a controversial factor, Da-Silva et al. (1998) found black race as a risk factor; however, Faisal-Curry et al. (2002) reported that white mothers are at higher risk for the development of PPD than black females.

Latino Women in the USA

Howell et al. (2005) found several risk factors including: maternal age less than 25 year-old, low educational level, a child suffering from colics, having a poor social support, physical symptoms and functional limitations, feelings of decreased self-efficiency in managing the infant and household affairs, and having limited access to health services.

Martinez-Schallmoser et al. (2003), found several factors similar to those previously described and specifically sought correlations between several variables related to acculturation, social support, quality of life, and depression. Key findings involved social/cultural factors related to antenatal depression, and that during the postpartum period a greater conflict with the mother's social network was related to dissatisfaction with postpartum support, particularly from their husbands or partners ($r= -0.38$, $p< 0.05$).

Significant predictors of postpartum depression in Hispanic mothers according to Beck et al. (2005) were Puerto Rican ethnicity, cesarean delivery, and being single.

Freeman et al. (2005) studying a sample of women predominantly Hispanic (53.2%) identified smoking and family mental health problems as risk factors for high EPDS scores.

Heilemann et al. (2004) studied women of Mexican descent and found that postpartum depression inversely correlated with mastery, satisfaction with life, personal competence acceptance of self and life, and importance of spiritual beliefs. A relation between "exposure to USA in childhood" and "higher depressive symptoms" was also found in childbearing (pregnant and postpartum) women, thus, women who spent their childhood in Mexico had lower levels of depression.

MOTHERS AND THEIR CHILDREN: THE IMPACT OF POSTPARTUM DEPRESSION

A study regarding the relationship between PPD and child-care (Medeiros & Furtado, 2004) was conducted in Brazil comparing the care provided by mothers with depression (n=10) and without it (n=12). Results showed that PPD was linked to events suggestive of maternal negligence and lack of breast-feeding. Hence, mothers with higher numbers of events suggestive of negligence (e.g. episodes of fever, skin irritation, colics, accidents, forgetting to give prescribed medications) presented with EPDS scores significantly higher than those of mothers with lower incidents of such events (EPDS score 18.2 vs. 9.7, $p<0.05$).

Mothers providing exclusively breast-feeding to their children had significantly lower EPDS mean scores than those that were no longer exclusively breast-feeding (p<0.05).

As discussed in a previous section, premature birth seems to be an associated risk factor; consequently a study in Argentina reported a specific intervention with mothers of premature children (Ruiz et al., 2005) targeted to the needs of the child and their parents, their parenting abilities, and factors that may interfere with child-care and safety. Mothers of premature children included in a program developed by Lester and collaborators (1996), showed levels of stress and depression significantly lower than a control group who did not receive the intervention. The mean score of the BDI, used to assess depression, was 9.0 in the group of mothers participanting in the program versus 19.6 in the control group.

CONCLUSION

Studies in Latino-America reported a prevalence of postpartum depressive symptomatology that varies between 5.92% and 48%; evaluations were usually conducted with previously validated assessment instruments in Spanish or Portuguese language.

A number of risk factors are consistent with the international literature, and involved a diversity of variables including: stressors, demographic and socioeconomic status, educational level, social and family support, relationship with partner, expectations about the pregnancy, number of previous pregnancies, newborn health, and maternal mental and general medical problems.

Depression, both maternal and paternal, may interfere with parenting abilities and the care and safety of the child, therefore appropriate interventions to diagnose, treat, and educate families is needed. Effective evaluation should not be limited to obstetric settings but must also involve multidisciplinary teams including pediatricians, nurses, psychiatrists, psychologists and primary care professionals in general.

REFERENCES

Alvarado M, R., Rojas C, M., Morandé, J., Neves G, E., Olea, E., Perucca, E., & Vera, A. (1992a). Cuadros depresivos en el postparto y variables asociadas en una cohorte de 125 mujeres embarazadas. *Rev. psiquiatr. (Santiago de Chile), 9(3/4)*, 1168-1175.

Alvarado M., R., Vera C., A., Rojas C., M., Olea, E., Morandes, J., & Neves, E. (1992b). La escala de Edinburgo para la detección de cuadros depresivos en el postparto. *Rev Psiquiatr (Santiago de Chile), 9(3/4)*, 1177-1181.

Alvarado M., R., Perucca P., E., Rojas, M., Monardes, J., Olea, E., Neves G., E., & Vera C., A. (1993a). Aspectos gineco-obstétricos en mujeres que desarrollan una depresión en el postparto. *Rev Chil Obstet. ginecol, 58(3)*, 239-244.

Alvarado Muñoz, R., Vera C., A., Monardes, J., Rojas, M., Olea, E., & Neves, E. (1993b). El inventario de depresión de Beck en los cuadros depresivos del embarazo y del postparto. *Rev Psiquiatr (Santiago de Chile), 10(2)*, 4-13.

Alvarado Muñoz, R., Vera C., A., Rojas, M., Olea, E., Monardes, J., Neves, E., & Perucca, E. (1994). Eventos vitales, soporte social y depresión en el postparto. *Rev Psiquiatr. (Santiago de Chile), 11(3)*, 121-126.

Alvarado, R., Rojas, M., Monardes, J., Perucca Páez, E., Neves G., E., Olea, E., & Vera C., A. (2000). Cuadros depresivos en el postparto en una cohorte de embarazadas: construcción de un modelo causal. *Rev Chil Neuro-psiquiatr, 38(2)*, 84-93.

Bandolier (1996): How Good is That Test II. Bandolier Evidence-based health care 27, 64-66.

Beck, C. T. (2001). Predictors of postpartum depression: an update. Nurs Res, 50(5), 275-285.

Beck CT, Bernal H & Froman RD (2003). Methods to document semantic equivalence of a translated scale. *Res Nurs Health 26(1)*, 64-73.

Beck, C. T., & Gable, R. K. (2003). Postpartum depression screening scale: Spanish version. *Nurs Res, 52(5)*, 296-306.

Beck, C. T., Froman, R. D., & Bernal, H. (2005). Acculturation level and postpartum depression in Hispanic mothers. *MCN Am J Matern Child Nurs, 30(5)*, 299-304.

Beck, C. T., & Gable, R. K. (2005). Screening performance of the postpartum depression screening scale--Spanish version. *J Transcult Nurs, 16(4)*, 331-338.

Betalleluz Pallardel, J. R., & Quiroz Valdivia, R. (1997). Sindrome de tristeza postparto hospitalario en la ciudad del Cusco. *SITUA, 5 (9)*:8-13.

Chaudron, L. H., Kitzman, H. J., Peifer, K. L., Morrow, S., Perez, L. M., & Newman, M. C. (2005). Self-recognition of and provider response to maternal depressive symptoms in low-income Hispanic women. *J Womens Health (Larchmt), 14(4)*, 331-338.

Coutinho, D. S., Baptista, M. N., & Morais, P. R. (2002). Depressão pós-parto: prevalência e correlação com o suporte social. *Infanto Rev. Neuropsiquiatr Infanc Adolesc, 10(2)*, 63-71.

Cox JL, Holden JM, Sagovsky R (1987). Development of the 10-item, Edinburgh Postnatal Depression Scale. *Br J Psychiatry 150*, 782-786.

Da-Silva, V. A. d., Moraes-Santos, A. R., Carvalho, M. S., Martins, M. L. P., & Teixeira, N. A. (1998). Prenatal and postnatal depression among low-income Brazilian women. *Braz J Med Biol Res, 31(6)*, 799-804.

Eizirik, L. S. (1984). Depressão puerperal: efeitos de prematuridade e risco de vida do recém-nascido no estado emocional da puérpera. *Ciênc Cult. (São Paulo), 36(6)*, 1002-1007.

Evans M., G., Vicuña M., M., & Marín, R. (2003). Depresion postparto realidad en el sistema publico de atencion de salud. *Rev Chil Obstet Ginecol, 68(6)*, 491-494.

Faisal-Cury, A., Tedesco, J. J., Kahhale, S., Menezes, P. R., & Zugaib, M. (2004). Postpartum depression: in relation to life events and patterns of coping. *Arch Women Ment Health, 7(2)*, 123-131.

Florenzano, R., Feuerhake, O., Hinrichsen, M., & Figueroa, C. (1984). La calibración de una escala cuantitativa para medir el nivel de depresión en poblaciones. *Rev Chil Neuro-Psiquiat, 22*, 17-23.

Freeman MP, Wright R, Watchman M, Wahl RA, Sisk DJ, Fraleigh L, Weibrecht JM (2005). Postpartum depression assessments at well-baby visits: screening feasibility, prevalence, and risk factors. *J Womens Health (Larchmt) 14(10)*, 929-935.

Halbreich, J., & Karkun, S. (2006). Cross-cultural and social diversity of prevalence of postpartum depression and depressive symptoms. *J Affect Disord, in press*.

Hasbún Hernández, J., Risco Neira, L., Jadresic Marinovic, E., Galleguillo U., T., González A., M., & Garay S., J. (1999). Depresión postparto: prevalencia y factores de riesgo. *Rev Chil Obstet Ginecol, 64(6)*, 466-470.

Heilemann, M., Frutos, L., Lee, K., & Kury, F. S. (2004). Protective strength factors, resources, and risks in relation to depressive symptoms among childbearing women of Mexican descent. *Health Care Women Int, 25(1)*, 88-106.

Howell, E. A., Mora, P. A., Horowitz, C. R., & Leventhal, H. (2005). Racial and ethnic differences in factors associated with early postpartum depressive symptoms. *Obstet Gynecol, 105(6)*, 1442-1450.

Jadresic Vargas, E., Jara V., C., Miranda, M., Arrau, B., & Araya, R. (1992). Trastornos emocionales en el embarazo y el puerperio: estudio prospectivo de 108 mujeres. *Rev Chil Neuro-psiquiatr, 30(2)*, 99-106.

Jadresic M., E., Jara V., C., & Araya B., R. (1992b). Depresión en el embarazo y el puerperio: estudio de factores de riesgo. *Acta Psiquiátr Psicol Am Lat, 39(1)*, 63-74.

Jadresic, E., Araya, R., & Jara, C. (1995). Validation of the Edinburgh Postnatal Depression Scale (EPDS) in Chilean postpartum women. *J Psychosom Obstet Gynaecol, 16(4)*, 187-191.

Jadresic Marinovic, E., & Araya B., R. (1995). Prevalencia de depresión postparto y factores asociados en Santiago, Chile. *Rev Méd Chile, 123(6)*, 694-699.

Kennerley, H., & Gath, D. (1989). Maternity blues. Detection and measurement by questionnaire. *Br J Psychiatry, 155*, 356-362.

Lester, B., Bigsby, R., High, P., Wu, S. (1996) Principles of intervention for preterm infant in the NICU. Presented at the 10 Canadian Ross Conference in Pediatrics. Optimizing the neonatal intensive care environment. 80.

Luis, M. A. V., & Oliveira, E. R. d. (1998). Transtornos mentais na gravidez, parto e puerpério, na região de Ribeirão Preto-SP-Brasil. *Rev. Esc. Enfermagem USP, 32(4)*, 314-324.

Martinez-Schallmoser, L., Telleen, S., & MacMullen, N. J. (2003). The effect of social support and acculturation on postpartum depression in Mexican American women. *J Transcult Nurs, 14(4)*, 329-338.

Medeiros, P. P. V. d. F., & Furtado, E. F. (2004). Perfil dos cuidados maternos em mães deprimidas e não-deprimidas no período puerperal. *J Bras Psiquiatr, 53(4)*, 227-234.

Miller, L. J. (1999). Introduction. In L. J. Miller (Ed.), *Postpartum mood disorders*. Washington, DC: American Psychiatric Press, Inc.

Moraes, I. G. d. S., Pinheiro, R. T., Silva, R. A. d., Horta, B. L., Sousa, P. L. R., & Faria, A. D. (2006). Prevalência da depressão pós-parto e fatores associados. *Rev Saúde Pública, 40(1)*, 65-70.

Moreno Zaconeta, A., Domingues Casulari Da Motta, L. l., & França, P. S. (2004). Depresión postparto: prevalencia de test de rastreo positivo en puérperas del Hospital Universitario de Brasilia, Brasil. *Rev Chil Obstet Ginecol, 69(3)*, 209-213.

O'Hara, M. W., & Swain, A. M. (1996). Rate and risk of postpartum depression. A meta-analysis. *International Review of Psychiatry, 8*, 37-54.

Pinheiro RT, Magallanes PV, Horta BL, Pinheiro KA, Silva RA, Pinto RH (2006). Is paternal postpartum depression associated with maternal postpartm depression? Population-based study in Brasil. *Acta Psychiatr Scand 113(3)*, 230-232.

Rohde, L. A., Busnello, E. A. D. A., Wolf, A. L., Zomer, A., Shansis, F., Martins, S. d. O., & Tramontina, S. (1998). Postpartum blues syndrome in Brazilian women: an investigation of associated factors. *Rev HCPA & Fac Med Univ Fed Rio Gd do Sul, 18(1)*, 42-49.

Ruíz, A. L., Ceriani Cernadas, J. M., Cravedi, V., & Rodríguez, D. (2005). Estrés y depresión en madres de prematuros: un programa de intervención. *Arch Argent Pediatr, 103(1)*, 36-45.

Santos, M. F. d., Martins, F. C., & Pasqual, L. (1999). Escala de auto-avaliação de depressão pós-parto: estudo no Brasil. *Rev Psiquiatr Clín. (São Paulo), 26(2)*, 90-95.

US Census Bureau. (2001). *The Hispanic population. Census 2000 Brief.* Washington DC: US Department of Commerce.

Vega-Dienstmaier, J. M., Mazzotti, G., Stucchi-Portocarrero, S., & Campos, M. (1999). Prevalencia y factores de riesgo para depresión en mujeres postparto. *Actas Esp Psiquiatr, 27(5)*, 299-303.

Vega-Dienstmaier, J. M., Mazzotti Suarez, G., & Campos Sanchez, M. (2002). [Validation of a Spanish version of the Edinburgh Postnatal Depression Scale]. *Actas Esp Psiquiatr, 30(2)*, 106-111.

Welch, B., Schafer, R., Dember, C.H. (1961). TAT stories of hypomanic and depressed patients *J Proj Tech 25*, 221-232

Wolf, A. W., De Andraca, I., & Lozoff, B. (2002). Maternal depression in three Latin-American samples. *Soc Psychiatry Psychiatr Epidemiol, 37(4)*, 169-176.

Wyszynski, A. & Lusskin, S. (2005). The obstetrics patient. In A. Wyszynski & B. Wyszynski (Eds.), *Manual of psychiatric care for the medically ill*. Arlington: American Psychiatric Publishing, Inc.

Chapter III

IMPLEMENTING UNIVERSAL SCREENING PROGRAMMES FOR POSTPARTUM DEPRESSION – POSSIBILITIES AND RISKS

Birgitta Wickberg[*]

Unit of Research and Development in Primary Care, South Bohuslän, Sweden.

ABSTRACT

Postpartum depression is the most common complication of childbearing with a prevalence of 10-15%, although there is a wide range of rates in different countries. The context and consequences of postpartum depression differs from depression during other times, as it may have negative long-term effects not only for the woman and her family, but also the mother–infant relationship and in turn the emotional and cognitive development of the child. Despite the more or less frequent contacts with health services after childbirth, women with depression often remain undiagnosed and untreated. Reliable, valid screening instruments have, however, been developed and psychological, as well as pharmacological, interventions, have demonstrated to be effective. As a consequence, screening programmes for postpartum depression have been introduced in primary health care services in several countries. Along with these approaches, the evidence base and the possibilities and risks of such programmes have been debated, and issues concerning how to best implement service changes in order to improve mental health in the perinatal period are currently being discussed.

INTRODUCTION

Over the last twenty years the interest in postpartum depression among researchers, clinicians and parents has increased substantially. Because of the potentially negative effects

---

[*] Correspondence concerning this article should be addressed to

that depression during this period can have on a mother, her infant and their relationship, prevention and treatment of postpartum depression is now regarded an important public health issue in many counties (Brockington, 2004). More recently, there has been a shift in focus, from the narrow concept of postpartum depression to a broader perspective, encompassing the whole range of mental health problems in the perinatal period, in this context defined as pregnancy and the first postpartum year (Austin, 2004).

The importance of postpartum depression is centred upon several issues. First, it is common. Depression accounts for the greatest burden of all mental health problems, and rates of depression are particularly high among women of childbearing age, especially among those with children (Murray & Lopez, 1996). In the postpartum period, the prevalence of depression is currently considered to be 10-15% in Western countries. There is, however, a wide range of reported prevalence rates due to cultural variables, differences in perception of mental health and its stigma, and differences in socio-economic environments (Halbreich & Karkun, 2006). Although the prevalence of mild to moderate depression does not seem to be higher in women after childbirth compared to non-childbearing women (Cox et al., 1993; O'Hara et al. 1990) there is an increased risk of women becoming severely mentally ill following childbirth, not only a risk of the rare puerperal psychosis, but also of severe depressive illness found in 3-5% of women (Oates, 2003).

Second, the context distinguishes depressions in the postpartum period from depressions at other times. The presence and demands of the developing infant makes it a sensitive period, when the ability to care for the baby may be interfered by mental ill health. There is evidence, which suggests that postpartum depression may negatively affect the quality of the mother-infant relationship and, in turn, the cognitive and emotional development of the child particularly if the depression is long-lasting and combined with social adversity and marital conflict (Murray & Cooper, 1997). Although the majority of postpartum depressions are self-limiting, resolving within some months of onset, for some women childbirth is a stressor that triggers the start of recurrent or chronic episodes of depressive disorder. Between one fourth to half of the women with postpartum depression have episodes lasting 6 months or longer, the most significant factor in the duration of the depression episode being the length of delay to adequate treatment (O'Hara, 1987).

Third, pregnancy and the first months after childbirth is a period when women usually have frequent contact with the health services and those who are at risk or suffer from depression or other mood disorders may thus be identified and helped. Regular visits at health examinations i.e. of the child provide a convenient structure for health promotion, counselling and simple medication (Bremberg, 2000). Without a structured approach such as a screening procedure, however, health professionals detect only about 50% of cases of postpartum depression in routine clinical practice (Hearn et al., 1998). While severe depressions in new mothers are often detected, less severe presentations can easily be dismissed as normal or natural consequences of childbirth or transient difficulties in the transition to parenthood period. Minor depression, however, is associated with significant disability because it is also associated with co morbid anxiety and other disorders (Presisig et al., 2001) and a significant number of minor depressions will over time convert to major depression (Maier et al., 1997).

SCREENING FOR PERINATAL DEPRESSION – WHAT IS THE EVIDENCE BASE?

The prevention of mental health problems in the perinatal period and their deleterious consequences is now regarded as a priority both professionally and politically in several countries. In some countries, i.e. in the UK, Sweden and Australia, practice in community primary care has been changed and screening programmes for postpartum depression (Cox & Holden, 2003; Sundelin & Håkansson, 2000) and perinatal depression (Buist et al. 2002) have been implemented in the health care services.

Theoretically, in order to implement a universal screening programme certain criteria should be met regarding the condition (it should be common and serious and it's natural history should be understood), the screening instrument (it should be simple, safe, precise and validated) and the treatment (it should be available and favourably influence the outcome). In addition, the screening programme should show evidence from randomised controlled trials of reduced mortality or morbidity with benefits of screening outweighing risks. It should be acceptable to public and professionals with adequate resources and informed consent, be cost-effective, and finally, have ongoing evaluation and quality-assurance strategies in place (Wilson & Jungner, 1968). The applicability in a health care context of these criteria, usually employed by medical screening committees, have, however, been questioned and the arguments for and against implementing universal screening programmes for postpartum depression, whether using strict screening criteria or screening as part of a broader programme, have been debated (Buist et al, 2002; Gaynes et al., 2005; Henshaw & Elliott, 2005; Oates, 2003).

Despite many attempts, no predicative tool used in the antenatal period has demonstrated adequate psychometric properties in predicting postpartum depression. There is, however, a strong case for advocating early detection and intervention of depression and anxiety in pregnant women as an important target in its own right (Austin, 2004). Depression and anxiety are as common in pregnancy as postpartum and recent studies have reported on their potential negative effects for the infant (Glover & O'Connor, 2002; O'Connor et al., 2002) There is an emerging consensus that the booking interview for maternity services must include questions about previous psychiatric history, with mental illnesses included in the same way as physical illnesses, and current mental health. For women with a past depression or who currently report or appear to be depressed, a depression questionnaire could be used (selective screening). A model of combined psychosocial evaluation i.e. a structured interview (Reid, 1998; Matthey, 2004) and a brief questionnaire within a broader antenatal interview could cover well-established risk factors for depression such as depression or anxiety during pregnancy, a previous history of depressive illness, recently experienced stressful life events and low levels of social support (Robertson et al., 2004).

There appears to be sufficient research evidence and support for use of a screening programme postpartum to increase recognition of mothers who are depressed or in risk for depression. Main arguments for the implementation of a universal screening programme for postpartum depression are:

- Postpartum depression is common with a pooled prevalence of 13% (O'Hara & Swain, 1996).
- It is associated with adverse child outcomes (Murray & Cooper, 1997). Although there is mixed endorsement for postpartum depression as a prevention target to improve child mental health, it seems important to prevent the depressions to become long lasting or recurrent (McLennan & Offord, 2002).
- A valid, reliable screening tool, the Edinburgh Postnatal Depression Scale (EPDS) is available (Cox et al., 1987). It has been translated and validated in at least 18 languages and is widely used (Cox & Holden, 2003). The scale should be used as part of a screening programme and the combination of the EPDS and an interview, including clinical assessment and professional judgement, should be adequate to decide on any subsequent intervention (Coyle & Adams, 2005). Other questionnaires e.g. the Postpartum Depression Screening Scale (Beck, 2000) have not been used extensively.
- Early remission can be achieved by a variety of treatment strategies, both health visiting and pharmacological treatment. In a recent Lancet review, Ian Brockington (2004) stated that treatment should be focused on depression and any underlying vulnerability, will always involve psychotherapy and may involve medication or other specific treatment. Thirteen randomised, controlled psychological intervention studies were summarized, all but one were beneficial (Brockington, 2004). Because women are often unwilling to use medication in the perinatal period for fear of child exposure, psychological or psychosocial interventions are especially suited for this time frame. Psychotherapy should thus be considered a first-line treatment, rather than an adjunction to medication treatment (Stuart et al., 2003). Counselling (listening visits) by health care nurses has been recommended as the first treatment for mild to moderate depression and for more severe depressions interpersonal therapy has proven effective. Medication could then be reserved for severe depressions that do not respond to psychological intervention (Stuart et al., 2003).
- Screening provides an opportunity to access large numbers of women and facilitate pathways to best care (Buist et al., 2002).

Main arguments against implementing universal screening for postpartum depression are:

- Lack of evidence about the acceptability of routine use of the EPDS, both in the women and the professionals using it (Shakespeare, 2005).
- Inadequate evidence regarding outcomes and cost-effectiveness.
- Risk of increasing inequities in care if the screening strategy is not addressing all women, including those from ethnic minorities. Additional resources for culturally acceptable translation and counselling facilities are necessary (Shakespeare, 2005).

PUTTING THEORY AND RESEARCH INTO HEALTH CARE PRACTICE

The process of integrating evidence-based strategies from research into clinical health care practice is not simple and involves several issues of concern. There are i.e. differences in health care systems and in cultural contexts that may influence the aims and the consequences of a screening programme for postpartum depression. One important issue to discuss is the focus of the programme. Should it be on all families and a broader range of psychosocial problems and distress rather than depression or anxiety per se or should it be on families with high risk of developing perinatal mental illness? Is identifying distress and minor depression acceptable or of benefit? Arguments for that are that long-lasting minor depressions rather than major depressions influence the development of the infant in a negative way (Luoma et al., 2001) and that more severe disorders in women may be prevented. This must, however, be balanced against the risk of overwhelming service capacity.

Another issue to be considered is how the theoretical perspectives of the health professionals will influence the screening procedure and the choice of treatment and support (Beck, 2002). Are there other theoretical perspectives such as psychological, societal and cultural approaches that are complementing the medical model? Is depression regarded a dichotomous or a continuous variable with a spectrum of severity and sub-types? Should the screening for postpartum depression be diagnosis or problem based and what would be the merits and risks of a problem-based approach to the screening and the treatment (Lee & Chung, 2005)? Finally, is there a risk for medicalizing problems and distress that are "normal" and transient in the time of transition to parenthood?

Before universal "screening" is introduced, either through a screening measure like the EPDS, combined with an interview or an assessment through personal interviewing, the health care staff needs to be confident that resources are there for the mother/family and themselves throughout the whole screening process (Barnett et al., 2005). Firstly, and may be most important, pathways to care must be established and interventions need to build on cultural beliefs and practices. Other important resources that are needed are training, regular support and supervision for the health care personals, and clear guidelines describing the screening procedure, like i.e. the guidelines in Scotland (SIGN, 2002) and in Sweden (National Institute of Health, 2003).

Training of health care professionals is critical to the success of screening (Elliott et al., 2001) and simply making the EPDS available to health visitors will not improve the detection of depression (Murray et al., 2004). It is the quality of the interaction between the health professional and the woman in the screening procedure, that defines what is "sensitive" screening. The training should include a broader perspective on perinatal mental health and training in "listening" skills. It is also important to ensure that the professionals involved are able to deal sensitively with distress and refer appropriate (Buist et al., 2002). Some women will not accept help (referral) even when they are depressed and others do not need referral but may benefit from support and empathetic listening offered by the health care nurse. Ethical responsibilities i.e. how to inform the patient properly and how to ensure that the intervention offered is effective, are other important issues in a training programme. The recording of information about depressed women after clinical assessment must be clear and addressed properly in the training. Finally, the training should be updated regularly and repeated for new staff.

The importance of getting adequate support such as ongoing supervision/consultation to health professionals working with depressed mothers has been pointed out in several papers (Elliott et al. 2001; Murray et al., 2004). In a recent survey to a random sample of all child health nurses in Sweden, a majority regarded regular supervision in their work with postpartum depression as necessary to start routine screening with the EPDS. (Massoudi, personal communication).

The notion of "testing" or screening using a questionnaire is not a universal one and both screening programmes and interventions need to be culturally adopted, that is recognize and build on cultural beliefs and practices and adopt to the local health care system. Lee & Chung (2005) has pointed out that in developing countries many obstacles to improving the detection and treatment of postpartum depression are also applicable to psychiatry at large and that the work to reduce stigma, improve funding, educate the public and engage the policy makers to understand that investing in mental health care is strengthening the population as a whole.

POSSIBILITIES AND RISKS WITH A UNIVERSAL SCREENING PROGRAMME

Besides the expected effects of a universal screening programme for postpartum depression, such as improved rates of detection of depressed mothers and improved clinical outcome, there may be other possible spin–off effects. A structured method, as has been pointed out by Cox and Holden (2003), may give women permission to speak and give the health professionals permission to listen. Hopefully, this may lead to generalized gains for the health care practice such as improved relationship with parents and increased professional satisfaction (Fuggle & Haydon, 2000). Using structured methods, such as a screening scale, may decrease the risk for parents need for support/intervention being defined according to the interest, competence and work load of the individual health care professional (Wickberg, 2000). The use of a questionnaire could also be helpful in drawing attention of both mothers and health care professionals to issues of mental health. In a longer term, a screening programme for postpartum depression might change the focus of the child health services from the infant to the family, from physical needs to also include emotional needs, including the parent's mental health. Using the EPDS as a base for careful interviewing i.e. about issues related to stress, vulnerability, social adversity, as well as support and resources could be helpful in planning early interventions (Wickberg, 2000). In a large, national study, Swedish mothers seemed to be satisfied with the attention given to their infants at the child health clinics, but one third felt that their own needs were neglected (Örtengren, 2005). This study supported the current development toward screening for postpartum depression at the child health clinics in Sweden.

There are also risks imbedded in a screening programme including the EPDS that need to be considered. A review of 18 validation studies of the EPDS suggested a lower positive predictive value in a normal population than in the validation study samples. Many women without depression might be falsely identified as depressed, making a clinical verification of the diagnosis essential (Eberhard-Gran et al., 2001). A "false positive" means that the duration or level of depressive symptoms does not fulfil the psychiatric criteria for a diagnosis of depression. There is a risk of false positives being misdiagnosed, as the EPDS is usually used just once. In the original paper by Cox and colleagues (1987) a two-step procedure (the first screening being followed by a second after a few weeks) was recommended to avoid this problem. In clinical practice, however, health visitors have found it unethical to let the woman wait several weeks for treatment or support. Instead, the second screening has been replaced by a follow-up interview by the health visitor immediately after the first screening. Women with distress should be offered support and accurate diagnosis should follow. If the EPDS is described and used as a screening tool, not as a diagnostic tool, and carefully followed up by an interview, the risk of women who score as a "false positive" to become anxious could be overcome.

Other questions of concern are the best time point(s) for screening and if there should be one or several screening time points. Is there a risk to miss the estimated 3-5% women with severe depressive illness, because these are presented before the EPDS is commonly used (6-10 weeks postpartum) and their symptom profile is not covered by the EPDS (Oates, 2003)? In health care services case finding should be a continuous process and not a "once-for-one" project (Hall, 1996).

Cautions should be taken around false negatives. These could consist of women whose symptoms are not included in the scale. A French study has reported that the EPDS performs better with women who have depression and anxiety and will miss women with retarded depression (Guedeney, 2000). The false negatives could also include women who do not want to represent their feelings accurately on a self-rating scale, due to a variety of reasons, both on structural and personal levels. In addition, expressions of depression are culturally bound. In cultures where depression may be presented with somatic complaints the absence of somatic depressive items in the EPDS might be a problem. These problems could be avoided with sound validation studies.

A screening program may open up areas of significant needs of distressed women and this could raise ethical concerns. It has been argued, however, that it is better to acknowledge needs and try to meet them rather than to deny them and thereby increase the risk for negative long-term consequences. In an Australian article, Buist and colleagues (2002) argued that informing women about available resources, even if scarce, is empowering rather than unethical and that the stigma of mental illness will not be overcome by ignoring it's existence.

EVALUATION STUDIES ARE NEEDED

The evidence base for routine screening for postpartum depression has been debated, especially in the UK, where the National Screening Committee (NSC) initially recommended against screening for postpartum depression as well as against using the EPDS. The main reasons were lack of resources to provide adequate treatment for depressed women and lack of applicability of screening women from different cultures. After strong reactions by the health care professionals, however, the NSC recommended the EPDS to be used as a checklist only together with professional judgment and clinical interview (Shakespeare, 2005) which was also the recommendation by Cox and colleagues for using the scale.

There are several studies going on trying to evaluate outcomes of screening for postpartum depression. In Australia, a three-year research programme, the National Postnatal Depression Prevention and Early Intervention Program (beyond blue) is evaluating outcomes of screening in terms of acceptability, cost-effectiveness, access and satisfaction with management in up to 100 000 women across five states (Buist et al., 2002). In Sweden, where the National Council for Medical Research has recommended implementation of postnatal screening and intervention throughout Sweden (Sundelin & Håkansson, 2000) an ongoing research program in two counties, "Changing Child Health Care", is evaluating the outcomes of screening with the EPDS (Sundelin et al., 2005).

In the UK, several evaluations have been done and some are planned i.e. the PONDER study in Sheffield commissioned by the National Health Service Research and Development Health Technology Assessment programme (HTA). The aim of this study is to compare two counselling interventions, non-directive and cognitive-behavioural counselling, delivered by health visitors in their usual clinical setting (Shakespeare, 2005). The economic costs of postpartum depression have been studied from a public sector perspective in a large high-risk British cohort. The study covered all aspects of health and social care provided to the mother and infant between delivery and 18 months postpartum. The mean cost differences between women with and without postpartum depression reached statistical significance for community care services (Petrou et al., 2002).

In USA, the US Preventive Services Task Force (2002) has recommended routine screening for depression in adult populations on the basis that the potential benefits outweigh the risks. It has established a three-stage framework for evaluating the effectiveness of screening that includes improved detection; increased referral or treatment utilization; and reduced morbidity (Harris et al 2001). Research on all three types of outcome is needed before the costs associated with screening can be justified and perinatal screening can be widely implemented as an evidenced based programme (Segre & O'Hara, 2005).

CONCLUSION

There is little evidence to date to support universal (routine) antenatal screening of all women for prediction of postnatal depression. Finding the best way of screening pregnant women, whether they are "at risk", have symptoms or a diagnosis of depression or/and anxiety is thus a research priority. Screening for depression in the postpartum period is likely to be useful because of the high prevalence of depressive disorders and the sufficient support for use of the EPDS. In addition, the evidence for the effectiveness of both psychological and pharmacological treatment seems to be sufficient to suggest that "best practice" methods are available (Buist et al., 2002). Research is, however, lacking regarding the cost-effectiveness and the acceptability to women and professionals of a universal screening programme. Before introducing screening, adequate resources must be available both for the women and the health professionals, such as clear pathways to care, adequate time resources, and training and regular supervision. One of the major challenges in implementing a screening programme in routine health care practice is that appropriate resources will be needed to address not only women with psychiatric diagnoses but also the whole range of psychosocial morbidity that will be detected, (Austin, 2004).

REFERENCES

Austin, M-P. (2004) Antenatal screening and early intervention for "perinatal" distress, depression and anxiety: where to from here? Arc Womens Ment. *Health. 7*, 1-6.

Barnett, B., Glossoop, P., & Matthey, M. (2005) Screening in the context of integrated perinatal care. In Henshaw, C. & Elliott, S. (eds.) *Screening for Perinatal Depression*, 68-82, London: Kingsley Publishers.

Beck, C.T. and Gable, R.K. (2000) Postpartum depression screening scale: development and psychometric testing. *Nurs. Res. 49*, 272-282.

Beck, C,T, (2002) Theoretical Perspectives of Postpartum Depression. *Am. J. Maternal Child Nursing, 27, 5*, 292-287

Bremberg, S. (2000) Quality of evidence for the present Swedish child health surveillance programme. *Acta Paediatrica 89*, Suppl. 434, 8-12.

Brockington, I. (2004) Postpartum psychiatric disorders. *The Lancet 363*, 303-310.

Buist A., Barnett, B.E.W., Milgrom J., Pope S., Condon J.T., Ellwood D.A., Boyce P.M., Austin, M-P. & Hayes, B.A. (2002) To screen or not to screen-that is the question. *MJA, Vol 177*, 101-105.

Cox, J. and Holden, J. (2003) *Perintal mental health. A guide to the Edinburgh Postnatal Depression Scale*. London: Gaskell.

Cox, J.L., Holden, J.M. & Sagovsky, R. (1987) Detection of postnatal depression: development of the 10-item Edinburgh Postnatal Depression Scale. *Br J Psychiatry 150*, 782-786.

Cox, J.L., Murray, D. & Chapman, G. (1993) A controlled trial of the onset, duration and prevalence of postnatal depression. *Br J Psychiatry 163*, 27-31.

Coyle, B. & Adams, C. (2005) The Edinburgh Postnatal Depression Scale: guidelines for its use as part of maternal mood assessment. In Henshaw, C. & Elliott, S. (eds.) *Screening for Perinatal Depression*, 212-216, London: Kingsley Publishers.

Eberhard-Gran, M., Eskild, A., Tambs, K., Opjordsmoen, S. & Samuelsen, S.O. (2001) Review of validation studies of the Edinburgh Postnatal Depression Scale. *Acta Psychiatr. Scand., 104*, 243-249.

Elliott, S.A., Gerrard, J, Ashton, C. And Cox, J. (2001) Training health visitors to reduce levels of depression after childbirth: An evaluation. *Journal of Mental Health 10*, 613-625.

Fuggle, P. & Haydon, K. (2000) Estimating resources for setting up an HV service for postnatal depression. *British Journal of Community Nursing, Vol 5, 7*, 348-351.

Gaynes, B.N., Gavin N., Meltzer-Brody S., Lohr K.N., Swinson T., Gartlehner G., Brody S.& Miller W.C. (2005) Perinatal depression: Prevalence, Screening accuracy, and Screening outcome. *Agency for Healthcare Research and Quality, Technology Assessment No 19*, ISSN 1530-440X.

Glover, V. & O'Connor, T. (2002) Effects of antenatal stress and anxiety: implications for development and psychiatry. *Br. J. Psychiatry 180*, 389-391.

Guedeney, N., Fermanian, J., & Kumar, R.C. (2000) The EPDS and the detection of major depressive disorders in early postpartum; Some concerns about the false negatives. *J Affect. Disord. 61*, 107-112.

Halbreich, U. & Karkun, S. (2006) Cross-cultural and social diversity of prevalence of postpartum depression and depressive symptoms. *J Affect. Disord.* E-pub, ahead of print.

Hall, D. (1996) *Health for all children. A programme for health surveillance.* 3rd ed. Oxford: Oxford University Press.

Harris, R.P., Helfand, M., Woolf, S.H., Lohr, K.R., Mulrow, C.D., Teutsch, S.M.and Atkins, D. (2001) Current methods of the U.S. Preventive Services Task Force: A review of the process. *American Journal of Preventive Medicine 20, 3*, 21-35.

Hearn, G., Liff & A. Jones, I. (1998) Postnatal depression in the community. *Br. J. Gen. Pract. 48*, 1064-1066.

Henshaw, C. & Elliott, S. (eds) (2005) *Screening for Perinatal Depression*, London: Kingsley Publishers.

Lee D.T.S. & Chung T.K.H. (2005) Screening in developing countries. In Henshaw, C. & Elliott, S. (eds.) *Screening for Perinatal Depression*, 90-98, London: Kingsley Publishers

Luoma, I., Tamminen, T., Kaukonen, P., Laippala, P., Puura, K., Salmelin, R. & Almqvist, F. (2001) Longitudinal study of maternal depressive symptoms and child well-being. *J. Am. Acad. Child Adolesc. Psychiatry 40*, 1367-1374.

Maier, W., Grnzyk, M.& Weifenbach, O. (1997) The relationship between major and subthreshold variants of unipolar depression, *J. Affect. Disord. 45*, 41 51.

Matthew,S., Phillips, J.,White, T., Glossop, P., Hopper, U., Panasetis, P.,Pertridis, A., Larkin,M. & Barnett, B. (2004) Routine psychosocial assessment of women in the antenatal period: Frequency of risk factors and implication for clinical services. Arc Womens Ment. *Health 7, 4*, 223-239.

McLennan, J.D. & Offord, D. (2002) Should postpartum depression be targeted to improve child mental health? J. Am. Acad. Child Adolesc. *Psychiatry 41:1*, 28-35.

Murray, L. & Cooper, P.J. (1997) *Postpartum depression and child development*. London: Guilford.

Murray, C.J.L. & Lopez, A.D. (1996) *The global burden of disease summary*. World Health Organization, Harvard School of Public Health & World Bank.

Murray, L. Woolgar, M & Cooper, P. (2004) Detection and treatment of postnatal depression. *Community Practitioner 77*, 13-17.

National Institute of Health (2003) *Postpartum depression* (in Swedish). Stockholm: FHI. ISSN 1651-8624.

Oates, M.R. (2003) Postnatal depression and screening: too broad a sweep? *British Journal of General Practice,* August 2003, 596-597.

O'Connor, T.G., Heron, J., Golding, J., Beveridge, M. and Glover, VV. (2002) Maternal prenatal anxiety and children's behavioural/ emotional problems at 4 years. *Br J Psychiatry, 180 (8)*, 502-508.

O'Hara, M..W. (1987). Postpartum "blues", depression and psychosis: a review. *Journal of Psychosomatic Obstetrics and Gynecology 73*, 205-227.

O'Hara, M.W. & Swain, A.M. (1996) Rates and risks of postnatal depression –a meta analysis. *International Review of Psychiatry 8*, 37-54.

O'Hara, M.W., Zekoski, E.M., Philipps, L.H. & Wright, E.J., (1990) Controlled prospective study of postpartum mood disorders: comparison of childbearing and nonchildbearing women. *J. Abnorm. Psychol. 99*, 3-15.

Petrou, S., Cooper, P., Murray, L. & Davidson, L.L. (2002) Economic costs of post-natal depression in a high-risk British cohort. *Br. Jpsychiatry, 181*, 505-512.

Presig, M., Merikangas, K.R.& Angst, J. (2001) Clinical significance and comorbidity of subthreshold and depression and anxiety in the community. *Acta Psychiatr Scand. 104*, 96-103.

Reid, A.J., Biringer, A., Carroll, J.D., Midmer, D., Wilson, L.M., Chalmers, B. & Stewart, D.E. (1998) Using the ALPHA form in practice to assess antenatal psychosocial health. *CMAJ 159(6)*, 677-684.

Robertson, E., Grace, S., Wallington, T. & Stewart, D. (2004) Antenatal risk factors for postpartum depression: a synthesis of recent literature. *General Hospital Psychiatry 26*, 289-295).

Segre, L.S. & O'Hara, M.W. (2005) The status of postpartum depression screening in the United States. In Henshaw, C. & Elliott, S. (eds.) *Screening for Perinatal Depression*, 83-89, London: Kingsley Publishers.

Shakespeare, J. (2005) Screening: The role and recommendations of the UK National Screening Committee. In Henshaw, C. & Elliott, S. (eds.) *Screening for Perinatal Depression*, 21-33, London: Kingsley Publishers.

SIGN. Scottish Intercollegiate Guidelines Network. (2002) *Management of postnatal depression and puerperal psychosis. A national clinical guideline* (SIGN 60). Edinburgh: Royal College of Physicians.

Stuart, S, O'Hara, M.W. & Gorman, L.L. (2003) The prevention and psychotherapeutic treatment of postpartum depression. *Arch. Womens Ment. Health 6* (Suppl.2), 57-69.

Sundelin, C. & Håkansson, A. (2000) The importance of Child Health Services to the health of children: Summary of the state-of-the-art document from the Sigtuna Conference on Child Health Services with a view to the future, *Acta Paediatrica 89*, Suppl.434, 76-79.

Sundelin, C., Magnusson, M. & Lagerberg, D. (2005) Child health services in transition: 1. Theories, methods and launching, *Acta Paediatrica 94*, 329-336.

US Preventive Services Task Force (2002) Screening for depression: recommendations and rationale. *Annals of Internal Medicine 136*, 10, 760-764.

Wickberg, B (2000) The role of the Child Health Services in promoting mental health: an introduction. *Acta Paediatrica, 89*, Suppl. 434, 33-37.

Wilson, J.M.G. & Jungner, G.(1968) Principles and practice of screening for disease. *Public Health Papers No 34*.Geneva: World Health Organization.

Örtenstrand, A. & Waldenström, U. (2005) Mothers' experiences of the Child Health Clinic services in Sweden. *Acta Paediatrica 94 (9)* 1285-1294.

Chapter IV

BARRIERS TO POSTPARTUM DEPRESSION SCREENING, DIAGNOSIS AND TREATMENT

Dean A. Seehusen[1], and Gary Clark[2]*

[1]Department of Family and Community Medicine, Eisenhower Army Medical Center Fort Gordon, GA 30809;
[2]Department of Family Medicine, Madigan Army Medical Center Fort Lewis, WA 98431.

ABSTRACT

Postpartum depression is the most common psychiatric condition experienced by women during the first year after the birth of a child. Postpartum depression continues to be highly under-recognized and under-treated despite a recent increase in public and professional interest. There are many barriers to proper screening, diagnosis and treatment that help to explain this trend. Patient barriers include a lack of knowledge about constitutes "normal" feelings in the postpartum period, a lack of knowledge about where to turn for help, fear of stigmatization and fear of using antidepressant treatment while breastfeeding. Provides barriers include a lack of knowledge about the frequency or severity of postpartum depression, a lack of knowledge that validated screening tools exist, uncertainty about how to treat identified women, fear of prescribing antidepressants to lactating women, a lack of time to screen and diagnose, and a lack of financial compensation for diagnosis and treatment. Recent research has looked at these barriers and suggests possible ways of overcoming them.

---

[*] Correspondence concerning this article should be addressed to:
Dean A. Seehusen, MD, MPH, FAAFP Research Director Department of Family and Community Medicine, Eisenhower Army Medical Center Fort Gordon, GA 30809. E-mail: dseehusen@msn.com.
Gary Clark, MD, MPH Director, Family Medicine Residency Program, Department of Family Medicine Madigan Army Medical Center Fort Lewis, WA 98431. E-mail: gary.clark@nw.amedd.army.mil.

INTRODUCTION

Postpartum Depression (PPD) has repeatedly been shown to be one of the most common conditions women suffer from in the months following childbirth [1]. Yet there is significant evidence that the condition continues to be highly under-recognized and under-treated [2,3]. Potential barriers to the diagnosis and treatment of postpartum depression have long been identified. Only recently, however, has research been conducted on these barriers. This chapter will review the previously identified barriers and the new research that has shed light on some of them. It has become increasingly recognized that pregnancy itself represents a period of increased incidence of depression [4,5,6]. Some authors have used the terms peripartum or perinatal depression to represent depression during or after pregnancy. For simplicity, this chapter will focus on postpartum depression but most of the barriers discussed apply equally to depression during pregnancy.

Barriers to postpartum depression screening, diagnosis and treatment can broadly be broken down into two categories: patient barriers and physician barriers. For both patients and providers, knowledge deficits represent the most important type of barrier and, therefore, those barriers that are most likely to be overcome.

PATIENT BARRIERS

The first barrier for patients is recognizing that they have a problem. Many women do not realize that the symptoms they are having represent an abnormal state and therefore it does not occur to them to seek medical help [7]. Coates et al. found that 75% of women with PPD felt that the symptoms they were experiencing were normal and only 28% had ever discussed their symptoms with a health care provider [1]. The mistaken belief that the symptoms of postpartum depression are normal may be supported by friends or relatives who recount having had similar symptoms during the postpartum period. Misunderstanding about what constitutes "normal" during this period is further compounded by the fact that symptoms such as fatigue and lack of concentration really are normal for new mothers [3,8].

Additionally, a majority of postpartum women suffer from "baby blues" and may be correctly informed that this is an expected condition and is not unusual. The "baby blues" are a self-limited period of emotional liability that does not extend beyond 10 days postpartum [7]. Women may not understand that emotional disturbances later in the postpartum period are a separate issue for which help is available.

Those women that do realize that what they are experiencing is abnormal still may not seek help. Mental illness continues to be associated with a significant amount of social stigmata [1,9]. Some women may avoid diagnosis out of fear of being labeled as having a mental illness [10]. Motherhood is touted as a joyous time in a woman's life. It is difficult for some women to admit that they are anything but happy and may perceive this to mean that they are in some way inadequate [7].

For one or more of the reasons cited above, the great majority of women with postpartum depression do not seek help. The studies conducted to date have shown that between 0 and 33% of women with postpartum mood disorders actively seek medical attention [1]. Women may attend their postpartum gynecologic visits and not mention their symptoms or they may skip the appointment altogether.

Those women who do desire treatment for their symptoms may not know where to turn for help. The peak incidence of postpartum depression is around 3 to 4 months after delivery [8]. Most women have their postpartum gynecologic examination completed by 6 to 8 weeks after delivery and may not have a follow-up scheduled for another year. This helps to explain why Coates found that most diagnosed cases of postpartum depression were diagnosed within the first month after delivery. The further out from delivery a woman gets, the less chance her postpartum depression will be diagnosed [1].

After their follow-up gynecologic examination, the only contact most women will have with medical providers during the first postpartum year is at their baby's well child examinations [11]. The concept of pediatricians screening for postpartum depression has not caught on widely so diagnosis at these visits is unlikely [12]. Even the number of exposures to pediatric care providers may be reduced because depressed mothers are less likely to adhere to recommended well-child care [3,13].

Concern about the safety of treatment for postpartum depression is a particularly difficult barrier for new mothers [1]. Selective Serotonin Reuptake Inhibitors (SSRIs), along with individual counseling, have become standard initial therapy for depression in the postpartum period [14]. The great majority of evidence suggests that SSRIs are safe in both pregnancy and lactation, but significant concerns on the part of mothers remain. Appleby et al. reported that over half of patients approached for enrollment in a controlled trial of fluoxetine for postpartum depression declined due to concerns about the safety [15].

In reality, infant exposure to antidepressants via breast milk is minimal and the risk to benefit ratio clearly favors treatment [4]. Most experts recommend making a decision on a case by case basis and not hesitating to use medications in postpartum depression because there is strong evidence that having an untreated depressed mother does adversely affect development. Children of mothers with untreated depression have been shown to exhibit cognitive delays up to at least age five [2]. Maternal-child interactions are significantly negatively impacted by maternal depression [3]. O'Brien et al. found postpartum depression in 21.4% among mothers of infants with failure to thrive versus 11.1% among controls [16].

PROVIDER BARRIERS

Like patients, provider knowledge deficits about postpartum depression represents a substantial set of barriers for screening, diagnosis and treatment [17]. This is true despite the growth of professional literature on the subject in recent years. A Medline search of the terms postpartum or postnatal depression on January 1, 2006 yielded over 500 results from the previous two years alone. Postpartum depression has become a popular topic for continuing medical education conferences and literature [12].

As a result, physicians are receiving some training on postpartum depression and most providers offering postpartum care now recognize mood disturbance as a serious complication of childbirth. In a study of over 300 actively practicing family physicians in the state of Washington, Seehusen et al. found that 90.2% felt that postpartum depression was a serious enough condition to warrant screening and 87.5% believed it was common enough to warrant screening [18]. Older physicians, further out from residency training are unlikely to have received training on PPD during residency, and are more likely to view postpartum depression negatively [18,19]

Beliefs about postpartum depression strongly affect screening practices. In the study by Seehusen et al., 77.7% of the providers who agreed that postpartum depression is common enough to warrant screening frequently screened for it at postpartum gynecologic visits. Only 18.9% of those who did not agree that postpartum depression is common enough to warrant screening were frequent screeners. Similarly, 73.9% of those who agreed postpartum depression is serious enough to warrant screening were frequent screeners while only 37.9% of those who did not agree were frequent screeners [18].

Those providers who recognize postpartum depression as a serious clinical entity may not realize that formal screening is mandatory to uncover most cases. When formal screening methods are not used, detection rates can be a low as 2%. Regardless of the specialty of the provider, usually less than 1/3 of cases are detected without a concerted screening effort [1,11]. Some physicians do not realize that reliable, validated tools for screening exist [19]. Seehusen et al. found that among Washington State family physicians who reported screening for postpartum depression at least occasionally, only 30.6% reported using a validated tool. A mere 5.5% of those who screened at least occasionally reported using a tool that was designed specifically for postpartum depression [18]. None of over 500 pediatricians surveyed in 2002 used a formal screening method to detect depression in their practices [12].

The most well studied of these tools, the Edinburgh Postnatal Depression Scale (EDPS), has been available for almost 20 years, has been validated repeatedly and in many languages; yet is still highly under-utilized. The EDPS is an excellent screening tool that has been found to be 88% sensitive, 92.5% specific in community samples [2]. The positive predictive value varies with the cutoff score used, but has consistently been found to be 70-90% even with the higher cutoff score of 12 [9]. The EDPS has also been validated for use during pregnancy [20]. Several other existing tools have also been validated such as the Postpartum Checklist (Beck, 1995) and the Postpartum Depression Screening Scale (Beck and Gable, 2000) [3]. Even a screening procedure as quick and easy as the 2-question depression screen is a reasonable option for postpartum depression screening [14]. This method has been found to be 97% sensitive and 67% specific for major depression in the general population [21].

Other providers are reluctant to screening because they believe that screening for postpartum depression is difficult, time consuming, and generally not worth the effort. Some may resist screening because they don't want to deal with the time consuming process of talking to an undiagnosed patient with depression. Seehusen et al. found that 19.2% of Washington family physicians felt that screening at every postpartum visit would take too much effort and 34.9% felt that screening mothers at every well child visit would take too much effort [18].

These negative beliefs translated into poorer screening practices. Among those physicians who believed that screening at every postpartum visit would take too much time, only 48.2% frequently screened for it versus 76.1% of those who did not believe that such screening would take too much time. Among those who believed that screening at every well child visit would take too much time, only 26.2% frequently screened versus 56.8% who did not believe it would take too much time [18].

Other providers may fear that screening for depression will be embarrassing or offensive to patients [22]. Studies have mostly found the EDPS to be acceptable for patients [9]. Interesting exceptions to this are a qualitative study by Shakespeare et al. which found many women did have some negative reactions to screening [10] and a study by Tam et al. in which only 7 out of 160 women approached agreed to participate in a screening study [23]. There are other providers who have frequent contact with postpartum patients who may not feel that it is their responsibility to screening, thereby wasting many opportunities for intervention. Only 57% of pediatricians surveyed in a 2002 study by Olsen et al. believed detecting maternal depression was one of their responsibilities [12].

Another set of barriers center around providers' feelings of uncertainty about treating PPD and fear of being held responsible for any bad outcomes [6,23]. Some providers may be uncertain if depression in the postpartum period needs to be treated differently than other depressions. This may be especially true of pediatricians, who until recently were receiving very little training on postpartum depression [3]. Only 31% of pediatricians surveyed by Olson et al. felt confident in their ability to diagnosed PPD and over half identified a lack of training as a barrier to their care of postpartum depression [12]. This is identical to findings by Wiley et al. [19]. It is easier for providers to not screen for and diagnosis postpartum depression than it is to deal with these uncertainties.

Many providers will be reluctant to use medications, especially as a first-line strategy. There is a generalized anxiety about treating women who are either pregnant or lactating with any medication [1,17]. This may be especially true of antidepressants which act on the neurologic system. The FDA has not approved any antidepressants for use during pregnancy [24]. There are scattered reports of adverse reactions in infants of mothers on SSRIs and it is recommended that starting doses be reduced by 50% in insure no side effects are noted [14]. It is also recommended that antidepressants be tapered near the end of pregnancy to reduce the risk of withdrawal-like symptoms in newborns [24]. About 2/3 of all reported cases of neonatal withdrawal syndrome have been with paroxetine [25].

Nevertheless, the consensus among experts is that these medications are generally safe and women should not be deprived of proper medical treatment simply because they are pregnant or breastfeeding. Instead, a frank discussion about the risks and benefits of pharmacotherapy should be had with the patient [24]. SSRIs are generally considered the first line agents due to their excellent safety profile [8]. Important neonatal outcomes are similar to infants not exposed to SSRIs in utero [26]. One Canadian study followed children exposed to SSRIs in utero for seven years and found no adverse effects [27].

Financial barriers to care for postpartum depression also exist. Reimbursement for mental illness screening and treatment is not comparable to screening and treatment of "medical" or "physical" ailments [1,28]. Many health plans do not included mental health care in the "postpartum package" of covered services [28]. Time is another manifestation of this financial barrier [20,8]. Olsen et al. found that over 70% of pediatricians found time to be a significant barrier to them diagnosing and treating postpartum depression. Another 29% noted insurance issues and 14% noted lack of reimbursement for treatment as barriers [12]. Taken together, these barriers create a serious disincentive because it is more time consuming and challenging to screening for, diagnose and treat mental illnesses, yet less financially rewarding. It is not hard to understand why a busy medical provider seeing a women for a routine postpartum gynecologic examination, or her child for a well child examination, would be reluctant to take the time and energy it requires to make a diagnosis which will invariably put him or her behind in clinic but for which he or she will not be adequately financially compensated.

OVERCOMING BARRIERS

Patient barriers will be most effectively overcome by education. Reports of a few well organized patient education programs have been published [29-31]. Several popular books have been published in recent years that have contributed significantly to public awareness of postpartum depression. These include personal accounts of PPD by Marie Osmond and Brooke Shields [32,33]. Several organizations exist exclusively for the education and support of women with postpartum depression. Depression after Delivery and Postpartum Support International are two such organizations [7]. Part of these organizations' mission is to educate prospective mothers, pregnant women and new mothers about the symptoms of postpartum depression and its therapy. The United States Military has developed a program called ISIS (Identify, Screening, Intervene, Support) that seeks to educate women and providers about depression during pregnancy and identify those at risk early [20].

Provider barriers will also take significant amounts of education to overcome. Residency is a particularly important time to train providers about postpartum depression [11]. The authors' own research has shown that residency education is highly associated with positive attitudes towards postpartum depression screening. Of those physicians who had received education about postpartum depression in residency, 74.7% were frequent screeners at postpartum gynecologic visits while only 35.5% of those who had not received such training were frequent screeners. After controlling for other significant variables, education about postpartum depression in residency was the strongest predictor of frequent screening in practice (OR = 8.1 for postpartum gynecologic visits, OR = 2.7 for well child visits) [18]. Education via the medical literature was also significantly associated with frequent screening [18].

These findings point to the need for structured educational programs designed to convey that postpartum depression is not overly burdensome to screen for, diagnose and treat. Over the last 5 years, Australia has implemented a nationwide educational program for postpartum caregivers [6,9]. In the United States, companies such as Danya International, Inc., are producing educational programs for medical providers. Danya's program, Support and Training to Enhance Primary Care for Postpartum Depression (STEP-PPD) is being designed specifically to improve training for primary care providers and their educators about these issues [34].

Any provider or practice that provides services for pregnant or postpartum women or infants should institute a reliable method of routine depression screening. It has been shown that such screening is feasible at routine postpartum gynecologic visits [1] and scheduled well child examinations [13]. Consideration should also be given to conducting such screening during pregnancy and at any contact with mothers during the first year after pregnancy [5,35]. Although there are several screening options available, as outlined above, the authors recommend the EDPS using a score of greater than 10 as the cutoff for further investigation into the possibility of depression [14]. It is important to also make sure a solid follow-up or referral plan is in place for those who screen positive [3,36].

Financial reforms that remove financial barriers to the diagnosis and treatment of postpartum depression will require legislative action in the United Stats. Individual medical providers and professional medical organizations should push for legislative reforms that require parity for reimbursement of mental illnesses [28].

CONCLUSION

Postpartum depression is a common and serious complication of childbirth. In recent years, the professional and lay literature have focused significantly more attention on the problem. Still, the disorder is widely under-diagnosed and under-treated. Recommendations that all new mothers be regularly screened have gone unheeded. Most providers who do screen rarely use validated screening methods designed specifically to identify postpartum depression. Those women that are diagnosed are often under-treated out of fear of medication use during lactation.

Numerous potential barriers have been identified that contribute to the current state of affairs concerning postpartum depression. More research is needed to give a full picture of which of these potential barriers most significantly impact the care of patients and how to overcome them. Knowledge deficits seem to constitute the majority of these barriers. In reality, this is good news because knowledge deficits can be overcome. Effective educational programs for both providers and patients plus improved financial incentives are important keys to widespread screening and better treatment of postpartum depression in the future.

The opinions or assertions contained herein are the private views of the author and are not to be construed as official or as reflecting the views of the Department of Defense

REFERENCES

[1] Coates AO, Schaefer CA, Alexander JL. Detection of Postpartum Depression and Anxiety in a Large Health Plan. *Journal of Behavioral Health Services & Research*. 2004;31(2):117-33.

[2] Cooper PJ, Lynne M. Postnatal Depression. *British Medical Journal*. 1998;316:1884-9.

[3] Chaudron LH. Postpartum Depression: What Pediatricians Need to Know. *Pediatrics in Review*. 2003;24(5):154-61.

[4] Haller E. Depression During and After Pregnancy: What Does the Primary Care Physician Need to Know? *Advanced Studies in Medicine*. 2005;5(1);21-6.

[5] Campagne DM. The Obstetrician and Depression During Pregnancy. *European Journal Obstetrics and Gynecology and Reproductive Biology*. 2004;116:125-30.

[6]   Buist A. Mental Health in Pregnancy: The Sleeping Giant. *Australasian Psychiatry.* 2002;10(3):203-6.

[7]   Seidman D. Postpartum Psychiatric Illness: The Role of the Pediatrician. *Pediatrics in Review.* 1998;19(4):128-31.

[8]   Clay EC, Seehusen DA. A Review of Postpartum Depression for the Primary Care Physician. *Southern Medical Journal.* 2004;97(2):157-61.

[9]   Buist AE, Barnett BEW, Milgrom J, Pope S, Condon JT, Ellwood DA, Boyce PM, Austin MPV, Hayes BA. To Screen or Not to Screen – That is the Question in Perinatal Depression. *Medical Journal of Australia.* 2002.177(Suppl);S101-5.

[10] Shakespeare J, Blake F, Garcia J. A Qualitative Study of the Acceptability of Routine Screening of Postnatal Women using the Edinburgh Postnatal Depression Scale. *British Journal of General Practice.* 2003;53:614-9.

[11] Heneghan AM, Silver EJ, Bauman LJ, Stein RE. Do Pediatricians Recognize Mothers With Depressive Symptoms? *Pediatrics.* 2000;106:1367-73.

[12] Olson AL, Kemper KJ, Kelleher KJ, Hammond CS, Zuckerman BS, Dietrich AJ. Primary Care Pediatricians' Roles and Perceived Responsibilities in the Identification and Management of Maternal Depression. *Pediatrics.* 2002;110:1169-1176.

[13] Chaudron LH, Szilagyi PG, Kitzman HJ, Wadkins HIM, Conwell Y. Detection of Postpartum Depression Symptoms by Screening at Well-Child Visits. *Pediatrics.* 2004;113:551-8.

[14] Wisner KL, Parry BL, Piontek CM. Postpartum Depression. *New England Journal of Medicine.* 2002;347(3):194-9.

[15] Appleby L, Warner R, Whitton A, Faragher B. A Controlled Study of Fluoxetine and Cognitive-Behavioral Counselling in the Treatment of Postnatal Depression. *British Medical Journal.* 1997;314:932-6.

[16] O'Brien LM, Heycock EG, Hanna M, Jones PW, Cox JL. Postnatal depression and faltering growth: a community study. *Pediatrics.* May 2004;113:1242-7.

[17] Gjerdingen D. The Effectiveness of Various Postpartum Depression Treatments and the Impact of Antidepressant Drugs on Nursing Infants. *Journal of the American Board of Family Practice.* 2003;16:372-82.

[18] Seehusen DA, Baldwin LM, Runkle GP, Clark G. Are Family Physicians Appropriately Screening for Postpartum Depression? *Journal of the American Board of Family Practice.* 2005;18:104-12.

[19] Wiley CC, Burke GS, Gill PA, Law NE. Pediatricians' Views of Postpartum Depression: A Self-Administered Survey. *Archive of Women's Mental Health.* 2004;7:231-6.

[20] Thoppil J, Riutcel TL, Nalesnik SW. Early Intervention for Perinatal Depression. *American Journal of Obstetrics and Gynecology.* 2005;192:1446-8.

[21] Arroll B, Khin N, Kerse N. Screening for Depression in Primary Care with Two Verbally Asked Questions: Cross Sectional Study. *British Medical Journal.* 20003;327:1144-6.

[22] Richards JP. Postnatal Depression: Postnatal Depression is not Being Missed in Primary Care. *British Medical Journal.* 1998;317:1658(letter).

[23] Tam LW, Newton RP, Dern M, Parry BL. Screening Women for Postpartum Depression at Well Baby Visits: Resistance *Archives of Women's Mental Health* Encountered and Recommendations. 2002;5:79-82.

[24] Lamberg L. Risks and Benefits Key to Psychotropic Use During Pregnancy and Postpartum Period. *Journal of the American Medical Association*. 2005;294:1604-8

[25] Sanz EJ, De-las-Cuevas C, Kiuru A, Bate A, Edwards R. Selective Serotonin Reuptake Inhibitors in Pregnant Women and Neonatal Withdrawal Syndrome: A Database Analysis. *Lancet*. 2005;365:482-7.

[26] Malm H, Klaukka T, Neuvonen PJ. Risks Associated With Selective Serotonin Reuptake Inhibitors in Pregnancy. *Obstet Gynecol*. 2005;106:1289-96.

[27] Nulman I, Rovet J, Stewart DE et al. Neurodevelopment of Children Exposed in Utero to Antidepressant Drugs. *Journal of the American Medical Association*. 1997;336:258-62.

[28] Sobey WS. Barriers to Postpartum Depression Prevention and Treatment: A Policy Analysis. *Journal of Midwifery and Women's Health*. 2002;47:331-6.

[29] Straub H, Cross J, Curtis S, Iverson S, Jacobsmeyer M, Anderson C, Sorenson M. Proactive Nursing: The Evolution of a Task Force to Help Women with Postpartum Depression. *MCN: The American Journal of Maternal-Child Nursing*. 1998;23(5):262-5.

[30] Hayes BA, Muller R, Bradley BS. Perinatal Depression: a Randomized Controlled Trial of an Antenatal Education Intervention for Primiparas. *Birth*. 2001;28(1):28-35.

[31] Spinelli MG, Endicott J. Controlled Clinical Trial of Interpersonal Psychotherapy Versus Parenting Education Program for Depressed Pregnant Women. *American Journal of Psychiatry*. 2003;160(3):555-62.

[32] Osmond M, Wilkie M, Moore J. *Behind the Smile: My Journey Out of Postpartum Depression*. New York. Warner Books, 2002.

[33] Shields, B. *Down Came the Rain: My Journey Through Postpartum Depression*. New York. Hyperion, 2005.

[34] Brown, Shana. Personal communication. January 31, 2005. This project has been funded in whole or in part with Federal funds from the National Institute of Mental Health, National Institutes of Health, Department of Health and Human Services, under Contract No. HHSN278200554095C. Available from Danya International, Inc. www.danya.com.

[35] Peindl KS, Wisner KL, Hanusa BH. Identifying Depression in the First Postpartum Year: Guidelines for Office-Based Screening and Referral. *Journal of Affect Disorders*. 2004;80:37-44.

[36] Gordon TEJ, Cardone IA, Kim JJ, Gordon SM, Silver RK. Universal Perinatal Depression Screening in an Academic Medical Center. *Obstetrics & Gynecology*. 2006;107:342-7.

Chapter V

PERINATAL DEPRESSION: TIME COURSE, SYMPTOMS, AND HORMONES

Alyx Taylor[1,3,*], *Vivette Glover*[1] *and M. Kammerer*[1,2]
[1]Wolfson and Weston Research Centre for Family Health, Institute of Reproductive and Developmental Biology, Imperial College London, London W12 0NN, UK;
[2]Hochschule für Angewandte Psychologie, CH 8032 Zürich, Switzerland;
[3] Thames Valley University, London W5 5AA, UK.

ABSTRACT

There is growing evidence that perinatal depression does not arise and develop in the same way for all women. We show here examples of how, for some, the symptoms start in pregnancy and resolve postpartum. For other women the symptoms are triggered by parturition itself. In a third group women experience a constant level of symptoms throughout. To enable research into the biochemical basis for these differences, the subtypes must be identified.

There is a large rise in plasma oestrogen, progesterone, corticotropic releasing hormone (CRH), and cortisol levels during pregnancy; cortisol, in late gestation, reaches levels found in Cushing's syndrome and major melancholic depression. Upon parturition levels of all these hormones decrease rapidly. Cortisol, oestrogen and progesterone all have strong psychoactive effects, and their sudden withdrawal may contribute to mood changes. It is possible that depression that starts in pregnancy more closely resembles the melancholic type associated with hypercortisolaemia, while depression that arises postpartum shows more of the symptomatology and hypocortisolaemia of the atypical type. Some women experience mild bipolar II depression postpartum, a subtype also associated with atypical symptoms. Different putative factors (genetic, hormonal and social) probably play a greater or lesser part in the etiology of postnatal depression in

---

[*] Correspondence concerning this article should be addressed to Alyx Taylor, Wolfson and Weston Research Centre for Family Health, Institute of Reproductive and Developmental Biology, Imperial College London, Du Cane Road, London W12 0NN, UK. Email: alyx.taylor@imperial.ac.uk.

different women. It is important to distinguish time of onset and resolution of perinatal affective disorder when investigating causal factors and symptom profile.

Keywords: depression, melancholic, atypical, antenatal, postnatal, cortisol

TIME COURSE OF PERINATAL DEPRESSION

The time course of depression in relation to childbirth is complex. For some, the symptoms start in pregnancy and resolve postpartum. While for other women the episodes are triggered specifically by parturition (Cooper and Murray, 1995). In a third group women experience a constant level of symptoms both during pregnancy and postpartum.

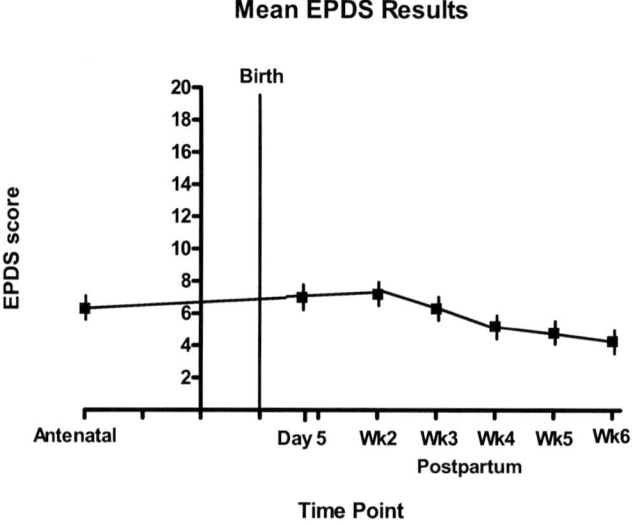

Figure 1a. EPDS results for the whole study. Mean with standard error bar for each time point. (n = 170)

A new study based at Queen Charlotte's Hospital, London was designed to investigate the development of symptoms of depression from gestation to 6 weeks postpartum. One hundred and eighty nine women attending the antenatal clinic were invited to take part in the study. They were asked to complete the Edinburgh Postnatal Depression Scale (EPDS) at 32 to 36 weeks antenatally, 5 days postpartum and then at weekly intervals until six weeks postpartum. The average age of the women participating was 30.8 years, with a range of 15-42 years. Of the 170 women who completed the EPDS at all time points, 15 (8.8%) scored ≥ 13 on the EPDS at 6 weeks. Figure 1a. shows the mean EPDS scores for the whole group. The EPDS scores peaked at two weeks postpartum, and had fallen to below the mean antenatal score by 6 weeks postpartum. The pattern for the whole group masked much individual variation. Figures 1b, 1c, 2a, 2b and 2c show examples of individual patterns of EPDS score. Twenty nine women (17%), had a very low EPDS score during the whole period (Fig. 1b). The largest group of women (49.5%) showed an increase in EPDS score postpartum that did not reach 13, and then subsided by 6 weeks. Twenty women (11.7%) scored EPDS ≥ 13 at 5 days or 2 weeks, which had subsided by 6 weeks (Fig. 1c). Thirty seven women (21.8%), had a raised EPDS score antenatally which had reduced by 6 weeks postpartum. Of the 15 women who scored ≥ 13 at 6 weeks, 4 (2.3%), had high antenatal scores (Fig. 2b), and 7 (4%), showed a sharp rise in the first two postpartum weeks (Fig. 2c). The EPDS scores of the remaining four women increased to ≥ 13 by week 6 postpartum, and the rise was either more gradual or erratic, so no typical pattern could be described.

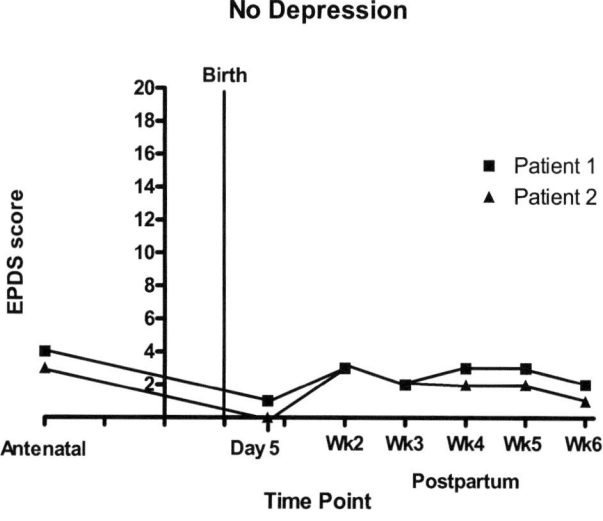

Figure 1b. Two examples where the EPDS score is 4 or less at all time points, representing no depression.

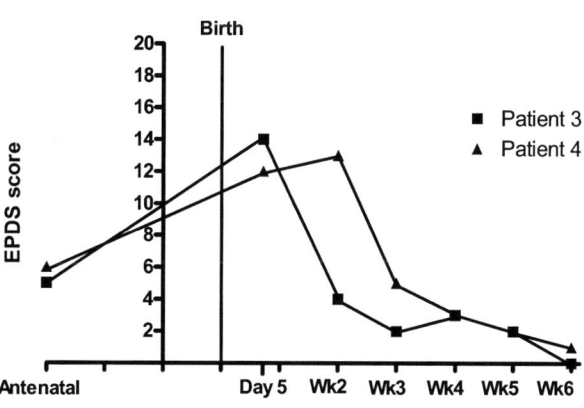

Figure 1c. Two examples where the EPDS score ≥ 13, on day 5 and / or week 2 and the decreases, representing transient symptoms of depression or severe blues.

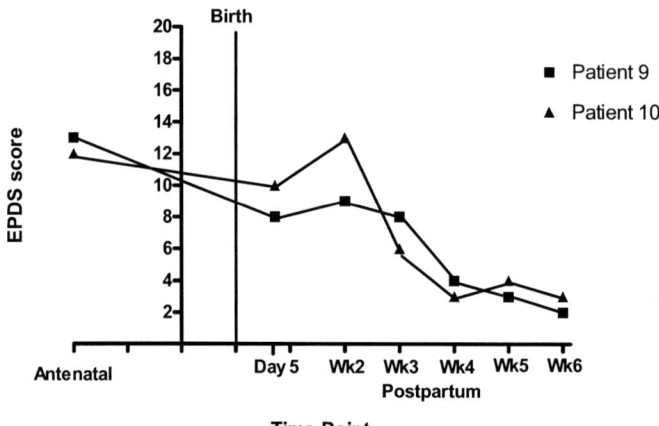

Figure 2a. Two examples where the EPDS score is ≥ 13, showing symptoms of depression antenatally, which then resolved postpartum.

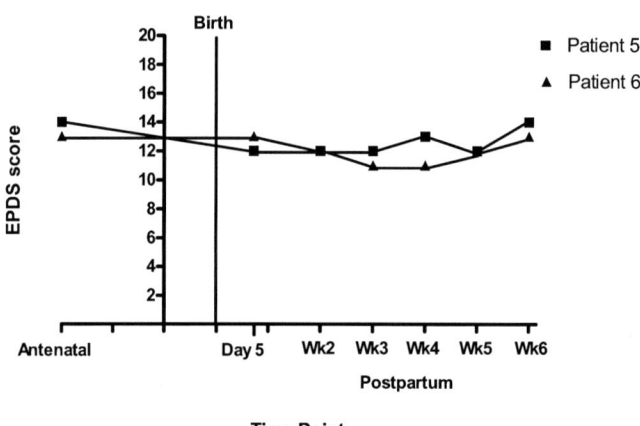

Figure 2b. Two examples of high and fairly steady scores at each time point showing constant depression.

The main finding of this study is that there are distinct subgroups of those women who scored EPDS ≥ 13 at 6 weeks. In some the disturbance of affect is present antenatally and continues postpartum at approximately the same level (Fig.2b). This is very different from the subgroup for whom the EPDS scores show a sharp increase in the early puerperium (Fig. 2c). It is therefore possible that underlying biochemical changes leading to these disturbances in affect are different in each subgroup of women.

Research and discussion of peripartum affective disorder still focuses most on postpartum depression. Nevertheless, there is now much evidence, including that presented above, that depressive symptoms are at least as common during pregnancy as postpartum

(Kitamura et al., 1996) (Evans et al., 2001) (Josefsson et al., 2001). In a recent study we have found that about 10% scored 13 or more on the EPDS at 8 weeks postpartum. This is similar to the findings of many other studies. However only about one third of these, or 3% of the total cohort, were depressed postpartum and not also depressed while pregnant (Heron et al., 2003). These studies have used the EPDS rather than a clinical interview, and more research into this area is warranted. However the evidence does suggest that a substantial proportion of women who are depressed after childbirth have been depressed in pregnancy also.

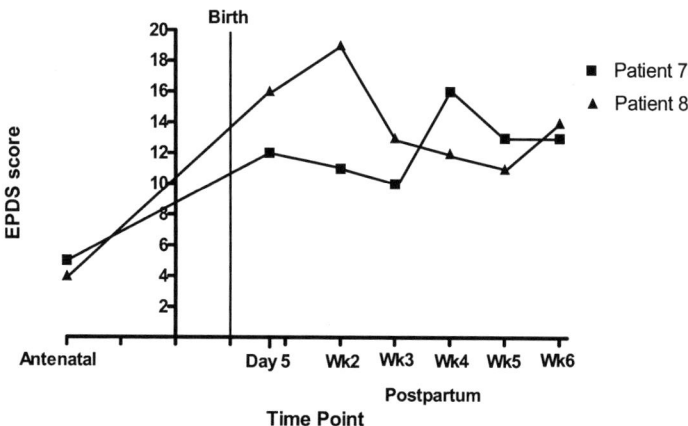

Figure 2c. Two examples of EPDS scores that show the development of symptoms of postnatal depression triggered by parturition.

Anxiety follows a similar pattern to depression with most women who are anxious postpartum also anxious while pregnant. In addition, anxiety during pregnancy is an extra risk factor for postpartum depression (Heron et al., 2003).

In order to understand the biological basis and pathophysiology of perinatal affective disorder it is essential to distinguish the time courses of onset and remission.

AFFECTIVE DISORDER THAT IS TRIGGERED BY PARTURITION - A CONTINUUM OF SYMPTOMS?

The group of disorders of affect that arise in the postnatal period include postnatal psychosis, the blues, the highs, and postnatal depression. It is well established that postnatal psychosis that affects about one in 500 women in the postpartum period is usually of the manic depressive type (Brockington et al., 1981), and that women with a history of manic depression are vulnerable to relapse in the postpartum period (Brockington, 1982).

At the other end of the spectrum is the blues, experienced by up to 80% of mothers, depending on which scale is used for measurement (Stein, 1980) (Kennerley and Gath, 1989). This is a period of lability of mood, crying, and headaches, that starts on about the 3rd day postpartum and peaks on days 3-5. Severe blues, or depression in the first postpartum week, are a risk factor for later depression (Kendell et al., 1981, Hannah et al., 1992, Glover et al., 1994).

Some women become over-elated postpartum (Glover et al., 1994); (Lane et al., 1997). This has been called the highs and is a mild form of hypomania. It has a distinct range of symptoms and a different time course from the blues, starting on the first postpartum day. It also is a risk factor for later depression. It has been suggested that there may be some shared biological mechanisms underlying this common but mild bipolar disorder and the rarer but more serious psychosis, which may be triggered at the same time (Glover et al., 1994).

Recently, the importance of co-morbid anxiety syndromes in the peripartum period has been stressed (Heron et al., 2003) (Matthey et al., 2003), but they have been little studied. It is increasingly recognised that some women suffer from posttraumatic stress disorder after childbirth and that the symptoms of this can persist (DeMier et al., 1996) (Ayers and Pickering, 2001, Callahan and Hynan, 2002, Soet et al., 2003).

Depression in general can be categorised into typical or melancholic depression, and atypical depression. Melancholic depression is characterised by loss of appetite and sleep, whereas those with atypical depression overeat and oversleep.

The blues, the highs, and bipolar psychosis are all triggered by parturition, and not by pregnancy. The postnatal syndromes are characterised by lability, mania or hypomania and depression of the atypical rather than melancholic type. Even though depressive symptoms are as common during pregnancy as postnatally, they are not associated with lability or bipolarity. It seems likely that the large hormonal changes that occur at parturition contribute to the postnatal spectrum of symptoms.

BIOLOGICAL CONTRIBUTION TO PERINATAL DEPRESSION

There is good evidence for several psychosocial risk factors for both antenatal and postnatal depression, especially the lack support of a partner or confidante (Warner et al., 1996), (Kitamura et al 1996), (Gurel and Gurel, 2000), (Hoffbrand et al., 2001). However the psychosocial factors do not account for all the variance and it is quite probable that there are biological causes also. The recent studies of Caspi et al (2003) have shown that it is only when one looks at a combination of life events and genetic vulnerability that one obtains an understanding of vulnerability of depression in general (Caspi et al., 2003). It is to be expected that vulnerability in the peripartum period will also be found to depend on both biology and environment, with different relative contributions in different types of disorder, and in different individuals.

GENETICS

There is good evidence for a strong genetic basis for puerperal psychosis (Jones et al., 2001, Jones and Craddock, 2001). Studies show a major overlap in the familial factors predisposing to puerperal psychosis and bipolar disorder. There is also evidence that familial factors play an additional role in vulnerability to the puerperal triggering itself. Jones and Craddock (Jones and Craddock, 2001) conducted a study of the occurrence of episodes of puerperal psychosis in families multiply affected with bipolar disorder, and found that puerperal episodes clustered in families. Episodes of puerperal psychosis occurred in 20 out of the 27 (74%) parous women with bipolar disorder who had a family history of puerperal psychosis in a first-degree relative but in only 38 of the 125 (30%) women with bipolar disorder with no such family history. These results demonstrate that familial, probably genetic, factors are implicated in susceptibility to triggering of puerperal episodes in women with bipolar disorder (Jones and Craddock, 2002).

The only gene polymorphism that has been identified so far in relation to peripartum mental illness is in the serotonin transporter (5-HTTT) gene. Coyle et al (2000) reported that variation at this gene exerts a substantial (odds ratio=4) and important (population attributable fraction=69%) influence on susceptibility to postnatal psychosis (Coyle et al., 2000). However this may not be a very specific effect, as variation in this gene has also been recently reported to reflect a vulnerability to non-psychotic depression in the general population, when considered together with life events (Caspi et al., 2003).

HORMONES

The HPA Axis

There are large changes in the levels of several psychologically active hormones over the peripartum period. Their evolutionary role is probably to help co-ordinate both parturition and the new maternal role of the mother (Carter et al., 2001). But in vulnerable women it is possible that these large hormonal changes also contribute to changes in affect, from mild mood disturbance to clinical depression.

The hypothalamic-pituitary-adrenal (HPA) axis is increasingly regarded as important in affective disorder (Checkley, 1996), (Tsigos and Chrousos, 2002). The most consistent findings in the biology of depression are that, as a group, sufferers have raised cortisol, and also fail to suppress cortisol output in the dexamethasone suppression test (Meyer et al., 2001). There is a strong interaction between the HPA axis and the female reproductive system, with glucocorticoids inhibiting pituitary luteinising hormone, and ovarian estrogen and progesterone secretion (Magiakou et al., 1997).

The function of the HPA axis changes considerably during pregnancy and postpartum (Magiakou et al., 1997, Kammerer et al., 2002). Corticotropin releasing hormone (CRH), which is normally only released from the hypothalamus into the portal circulation, and is not detectable in the plasma, is also generated and released into the blood stream, from the placenta. Plasma levels start to become detectable at mid gestation and rise exponentially towards term. Cortisol levels also rise greatly during pregnancy and, at the end, reach values comparable to those found in severe depression (Magiakou et al., 1997). This raises the question as to why most women do not feel depressed towards the end of their pregnancy. Cortisol levels drop postpartum, although taking some weeks until they reach normal values (fig. 3c). The dexamethasone suppression test, which is abnormal in most women during pregnancy, also takes some weeks to normalise (Owens et al., 1987) (Smith and Thomson, 1991).

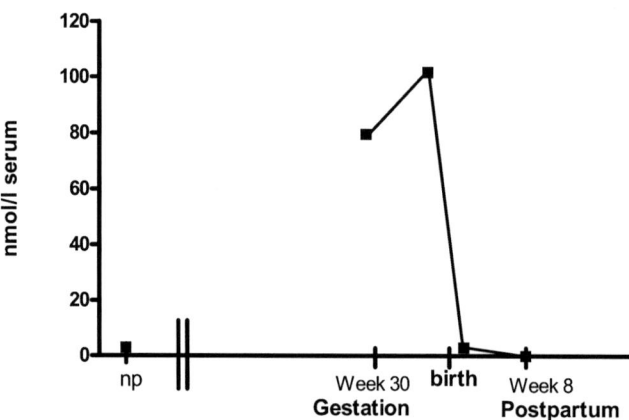

Figure 3a. 17β-Estradiol concentration in serum for non-pregnant women, at weeks 30 & 37 gestation and at weeks 1 & 8 postpartum (n = 40, for all points). Abbreviation np = non-pregnant. Based on data from Lommatzsch et al. 2006

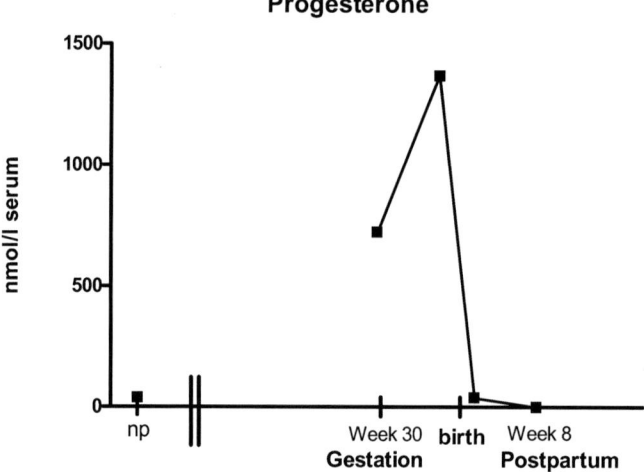

Figure 3b. Progesterone concentration in serum for non-pregnant women, at weeks 30 & 37 gestation and at weeks 1 & 8 postpartum (n = 40, for all points). Abbreviation np = non-pregnant. Based on data from Lommatzsch et al. 2006

It is possible that those women vulnerable to depression during pregnancy have different HPA axis function to those vulnerable to postpartum depression. We described earlier the contrasting symptoms of melancholic and atypical depression. These two forms of depression have also been found to have opposite disturbances in the HPA axis with melancholics showing raised cortisol and atypicals having lower than normal cortisol output (Gold and

Chrousos, 2002). One might expect that a vulnerability to melancholic depression would worsen during pregnancy, with a natural increase of cortisol, whereas those with a vulnerability to atypical depression might improve as the cortisol level normalised. Conversely those with a vulnerability to atypical depression might be more prone to postnatal depression. It is of interest that posttraumatic stress disorder, which can be triggered by parturition, is also associated with hypocortsiolaemia.

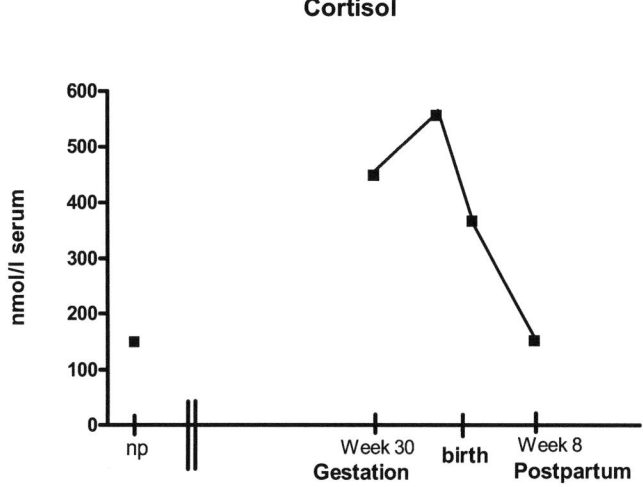

Figure 3c. Cortisol concentration in serum for non-pregnant women, at weeks 30 & 37 gestation and at weeks 1 & 8 postpartum (n = 40, for all points). Abbreviation np = non-pregnant. Based on data from Lommatzsch and co-workers (Lommatzsch et al., 2006).

There is as yet no evidence for this in relation to ante or postpartum depression. However, Magiakou et al (Magiakou et al., 1996) have shown that that the postpartum period is associated with suppression of hypothalamic CRH secretion. They followed the pattern of increase in plasma ACTH after a challenge with CRH in 17 healthy euthymic women starting at the 20th week of gestation, 7 women developed the blues and 1 developed depression. Overall, the mean plasma ACTH response to an intravenous bolus of 1 microgram/kg CRH was markedly blunted at 3 and 6 weeks postpartum but normal at 12 weeks. The mean plasma cortisol response was at the upper limit of normal at all 3 times. When the ACTH responses were analyzed separately for the euthymic women and those who had the blues or depression, the blunting of ACTH was significantly more severe and long lasting in the latter group. This was observed at all 3 times of testing. The authors conclude "that there is central suppression of hypothalamic CRH secretion in the postpartum, which might explain the increased vulnerability to the affective disorders observed during this period". It may be particularly marked in those with the blues, and those with severe blues are more likely to develop postpartum depression later (Glover et al., 1994). This pattern of suppressed CRH response is also similar to that observed in atypical rather than melancholic depression (Magiakou et al., 1997).

Significantly elevated levels of cortisol have been found to be associated with the blues (Okano and Nomura, 1992) (Taylor et al., 1994), and significantly lower levels characterised women who exhibited mild hypomania or the highs (Taylor et al., 1994) (Taylor et al., 1996). Low levels of cortisol were independently associated with epidural anesthesia, while elevated levels were related to assisted delivery (Taylor et al., 1994).

Estrogen and Progesterone

It is clear from animal models that the sex hormones such as estrogen and progesterone, which rise greatly during pregnancy, and then show a sharp drop immediately after parturition, have a great effect on the functioning of parts of the brain. They act on monoamine rich regions such as the locus coereleus and the raphe, which are known in turn to be involved in the control of mood. It is almost surprising that all women do not show greater mood changes at this time.

Estrogen and progesterone withdrawal are thus likely to play a role in the etiology of postpartum mental disturbance. They freely enter the brain and are known to interact with central monoamine neurotransmitter systems. However, studies which have examined levels of estrogen and progesterone in women with or without postpartum depression have generally proved negative (Wieck, 1989) (Bloch et al., 2003), although Harris et al have shown that women with the blues suffered a greater drop in progesterone form the ante to postpartum period (Harris et al., 1994). Some evidence for a hormonal component is given by the association of postpartum depression with other reproductive endocrine related mood disorders, especially the premenstrual syndrome (Sugawara et al., 1997). However studies in this area have been inconsistent.

Bloch et al (Bloch et al., 2000) have provided the best evidence, so far, for a role for sex hormones in the generation of postpartum depression. They investigated the possible role of changes in gonadal steroid levels by simulating two hormonal conditions related to pregnancy and parturition in non-pregnant women. The very high estrogen and progesterone levels of pregnancy, and withdrawal from these high levels postpartum, were induced in women both with and without a history of postpartum depression. The steroids were given for 8 weeks and then withdrawn under double-blind conditions. Outcome measures were daily symptom self-ratings and standardized subjective and objective cross-sectional mood rating scales. Five of the eight women with a history of postpartum depression (62.5%) and none of the eight women in the comparison group developed significant increases in depressive symptoms during the withdrawal period. Even though this was a small study, the authors plausibly conclude that these results do provide some direct evidence in support of the involvement of these hormones in the development of postpartum depression in a subgroup of women. It is likely that the susceptible women have a different sensitivity to the increase and/or withdrawal of these hormones rather than different levels of the hormones themselves (Rubinow et al., 1998). Table 1 summarises the biological findings in postnatal affective disorder.

Research into hormonal prophylaxis and treatment of postnatal depression and psychosis is limited. One recent review article (Karuppaswamy and Vlies, 2003) has explored the evidence available regarding the use of estrogen and progesterone. Although some early research by Dalton (Dalton, 1982), reported the benefit of progesterone in preventing postnatal depression, the studies were uncontrolled and have not been confirmed. Indeed, long-acting norethisterone enanthate (a synthetic progestogen) given within 48 hours of delivery has been shown to be associated with an *increased* risk of developing postnatal depression (Lawrie et al., 1998). There is some limited evidence that estrogen may be beneficial in treating severe postnatal depression (Gregoire et al., 1996), (Ahokas et al., 2001), and also in preventing its relapse (Sichel et al., 1995).

Table 1. Summary of biological findings in postnatal affective disorder.

Postnatal	Symptoms & Etiology	Biological findings	References
psychosis	Starts within 2 weeks	Genetic basis	(Jones and Craddock, 2001)
	Often of the manic depressive type	Increased growth hormone response to apomorphine	(Wieck et al., 1991) (McIvor et al., 1996)
	1/500 to 1/1000 births	Altered 5-HTTT gene	(Coyle et al., 2000)
	Recurrence rate high		
	Risk factor – family or personal history of manic depression		
blues	Starts approx day 3, peaks on days 3-5	Raised cortisol	(Okano and Nomura, 1992) (Taylor et al., 1994)
	Period of lability of mood, crying and headaches	Suppressed ACTH response to oCRH	(Magiakou et al., 1996)
	Experienced by up to 80% women		
highs	Starts of the first day postpartum	Lower cortisol	(Glover et al., 1994), (Taylor et al., 1994), (Taylor et al., 1996)
	Symptoms of hypomania including elation, racing thoughts and irritability		
Postnatal depression	Can be continuous with severe blues or arise separately	Greater sensitivity to increase and withdrawal of estrogen and progesterone in model trial	(Bloch et al., 2000) (Harris et al., 1989), (Harris et al., 1992), (Kuijpens et al., 2001).
	Risk factors: highs, blues or previous postnatal depression		
	Symptoms of atypical depression more common postpartum	Increased thyroperoxidase antibodies	
Postnatal post traumatic stress disorder	Flashbacks, difficulty sleeping, feeling detached or estranged May be chronic with symptoms increasing or decreasing	None	(DeMier et al., 1996)

As high rates of postpartum relapse occur in women with histories of bipolar disorder, and these relapses may be triggered by the post delivery fall in circulating estrogen, it is a reasonable hypothesis that estrogen administration after childbirth would prevent postpartum relapse. A recent study (Kumar et al., 2003) has tested this in 29 pregnant women with a diagnosis of hypomania, mania, or schizoaffective disorder in an open clinical trial, beginning within 48 hours after delivery. The study found that estradiol at all dose regimens did not reduce the rate of relapse, although there was a suggestion that those on the highest dose needed less other medication. The results did not support the original hypothesis and the authors concluded that the use of prophylactic estrogen in such circumstances is not warranted. However a small study of the effect of estradiol for the treatment of postpartum psychosis had more encouraging results (Ahokas et al., 2000), and this area deserves further study.

CONCLUSION

In the last ten years we have become more aware of the complexity of both ante and postpartum psychiatric disorder. Anxiety and depression are as common during pregnancy as after parturition. Some women suffer antepartum, some postpartum and some both. Postpartum psychosis, the blues and a mild hypomania, called the highs, can be triggered by parturition, as can posttraumatic stress disorder. Severe blues and highs are both risk factors for later depression. The postnatal syndromes are characterised by lability, mania or hypomania, and depression of the atypical rather than melancholic type.

Postpartum psychosis has a strong genetic component, probably including both a joint vulnerability with manic depression in general, and a specific vulnerability to a puerperal trigger. It is probable that the large changes in the psychoactive hormones cortisol, progesterone and estrogen that occur in the peripartum period play a part in causing psychiatric illness in some women at this time. We should be able to understand the biological components of these disorders more fully when studies are designed to differentiate the exact symptoms of each case (e.g. arising out of the highs), together with the time of onset.

ACKNOWLEDGEMENTS

Grateful thanks to Diana Adams for all her help with the studies at Queen Charlottes Hospital.

REFERENCES

Ahokas, A., Aito, M. & Rimon, R. (2000) Positive treatment effect of estradiol in postpartum psychosis: a pilot study. *J Clin Psychiatry, 61*, 166-9.

Ahokas, A., Kaukoranta, J., Wahlbeck, K. & Aito, M. (2001) Estrogen deficiency in severe postpartum depression: successful treatment with sublingual physiologic 17beta-estradiol: a preliminary study. *J Clin Psychiatry, 62*, 332-6.

Ayers, S. & Pickering, A. D. (2001) Do Women Get Posttraumatic Stress Disorder as a Result of Childbirth? A Prospective Study of Incidence. *Birth, 28*, 111-118.

Bloch, M., Daly, R. C. & Rubinov, D. R. (2003) Endocrine factors in the etiology of postpartum depression. *Compr Psychiatry, 44*, 234-46.

Bloch, M., Schmidt, P. J., Danaceau, M., Murphy, J., Nieman, L. & Rubinov, D. R. (2000) Effects of Gonadal Steroids in Women With a History of Postpartum Depression. *Am J Psychiatry, 157*, 924-930.

Brockington, I. F., Cernik, K. F., Schofield, E. M., Downing, A. R., Francis, A. F. & Keelan, C. (1981) Puerperal Psychosis. Phenomena and diagnosis. *Arch Gen Psychiatry, 38*, 829-33.

Brockington, I. F., Winokur, G. & Dean, C. (1982) *Puerperal psychosis in Motherhood and Mental Illness*, London, Academic Press.

Callahan, J. L. & Hynan, M. T. (2002) Identifying mothers at risk for postnatal emotional distress: further evidence for the validity of the perinatal posttraumatic stress disorder questionnaire. *J Perinatol, 22*, 448-54.

Carter, C. S., Altemus, M. & Chrousos, G. P. (2001) Neuroendocrine and emotional changes in the post-partum period. *Prog Brain Res, 133*, 241-9.

Caspi, A., Sugden, K., Moffitt, T. E., Taylor, A., Craig, I. W., Harrington, H., Mcclay, J., Mill, J., Martin, J., Braithwaite, A. & Poulton, R. (2003) Influence of life stress on depression: moderation by a polymorphism in the 5-HTT gene. *Science, 301*, 386-9.

Checkley, S. (1996) The neuroendocrinology of depression and chronic stress. *Br Med Bull, 52*, 597-617.

Cooper, P. J. & Murray, L. (1995) Course and recurrence of postnatal depression. Evidence for the specificity of the diagnostic concept. *Br J Psychiatry, 166*, 191-5.

Coyle, N., Jones, I., Robertson, E., Lendon, C. & Craddock, N. (2000) Variation at the serotonin transporter gene influences susceptibility to bipolar affective puerperal psychosis. *Lancet, 356*, 1490-1.

Dalton, K. (1982) The importance of diagnosing premenstrual syndrome. *Health Visit, 55*, 66.

Demier, R. L., Hynan, M. T., Harris, H. B. & Manniello, R. L. (1996) Perinatal stressors as predictors of symptoms of posttraumatic stress in mothers of infants at high risk. *J Perinatol, 16*, 276-80.

Evans, J., Heron, J., Francomb, H., Oke, S. & Golding, J. (2001) Cohort study of depressed mood during pregnancy and after childbirth. *BMJ, 323*, 257-260.

Glover, V., Liddle, P., Taylor, A., Adams, D. & Sandler, M. (1994) Mild hypomania (the highs) can be a feature of the first postpartum week. Association with later depression. *Br J Psychiatry, 164*, 517-21.

Gold, P. W. & Chrousos, G. P. (2002) Organization of the stress system and its dysregulation in melancholic and atypical depression: high vs low CRH/NE states. *Mol Psychiatry, 7*, 254-75.

Gregoire, A. J., Kumar, R., Everitt, B., Henderson, A. F. & Studd, J. W. (1996) Transdermal oestrogen for treatment of severe postnatal depression. *Lancet, 347*, 930-3.

Gurel, S. & Gurel, H. (2000) The evaluation of determinants of early postpartum low mood: the importance of parity and inter-pregnancy interval. *Eur J Obstet Gynecol Reprod Biol, 91*, 21-4.

Hannah, P., Adams, D., Lee, A., Glover, V. & Sandler, M. (1992) Links between early post-partum mood and post-natal depression. *Br J Psychiatry, 160*, 777-80.

Harris, B., Fung, H., Johns, S., Kologlu, M., Bhatti, R., McGregor, A. M., Richards, C. J. & Hall, R. (1989) Transient post-partum thyroid dysfunction and postnatal depression. *J Affect Disord, 17*, 243-9.

Harris, B., Lovett, L., Newcombe, R. G., Read, G. F., Walker, R. & Riad-Fahmy, D. (1994) Maternity blues and major endocrine changes: Cardiff puerperal mood and hormone study II. *Bmj, 308*, 949-53.

Harris, B., Othman, S., Davies, J. A., Weppner, G. J., Richards, C. J., Newcombe, R. G., Lazarus, J. H., Parkes, A. B., Hall, R. & Phillips, D. I. (1992) Association between postpartum thyroid dysfunction and thyroid antibodies and depression. *Bmj, 305*, 152-6.

Heron, J., O'Connor, T. G., Evans, J., Golding, J. & Glover, V. (2003) The Course of Anxiety and Depression Through Pregnancy and the Postpartum in a Community Sample. *Journal of Affective Disorders.*

Hoffbrand, S., Howard, L. & Crawley, H. (2001) Antidepressant drug treatment for postnatal depression. *Cochrane Database Syst Rev*, CD002018.

Jones, I. & Craddock, N. (2001) Familiality of the puerperal trigger in bipolar disorder: results of a family study. *Am J Psychiatry, 158*, 913-7.

Jones, I. & Craddock, N. (2002) Do puerperal psychotic episodes identify a more familial subtype of bipolar disorder? Results of a family history study. *Psychiatr Genet, 12*, 177-80.

Jones, I., Lendon, C., Coyle, N., Robertson, E., Brockington, I. & Craddock, N. (2001) Molecular genetic approaches to puerperal psychosis. *Prog Brain Res, 133*, 321-31.

Josefsson, A., Berg, G., Nordin, C. & Sydsjo, G. (2001) Prevalence of depressive symptoms in late pregnancy and postpartum. Acta Obstet Gynecol Scand, 80, 251-5.

Kammerer, M., Adams, D., Castelberg BV, B. & Glover, V. (2002) Pregnant women become insensitive to cold stress. *BMC Pregnancy Childbirth, 2*, 8.

Karuppaswamy, J. & Vlies, R. (2003) The benefit of oestrogens and progestogens in postnatal depression. *J Obstet Gynaecol, 23*, 341-6.

Kendell, R. E., McGuire, R. J., Connor, Y. & Cox, J. L. (1981) Mood changes in the first three weeks after childbirth. *J Affect Disord, 3*, 317-26.

Kennerley, H. & Gath, D. (1989) Maternity Blues : Detection and measurement by questionnaire. *British Journal of Psychiatry, 155*, 356-362.

Kitamura, T., Sugawara, M., Sugawara, K., Toda, M. A. & Shima, S. (1996) Psychosocial study of depression in early pregnancy. *Br J Psychiatry, 168*, 732-8.

Kuijpens, J. L., Vader, H. L., Drexhage, H. A., Wiersinga, W. M., Van Son, M. J. & Pop, V. J. (2001) Thyroid peroxidase antibodies during gestation are a marker for subsequent depression postpartum. *Eur J Endocrinol, 145*, 579-84.

Kumar, C., McIvor, R. J., Davies, T., Brown, N., Papadopoulos, A., Wieck, A., Checkley, S. A., Campbell, I. C. & Marks, M. N. (2003) Estrogen administration does not reduce the rate of recurrence of affective psychosis after childbirth. *J Clin Psychiatry, 64*, 112-8.

Lane, A., Keville, R., Morris, M., Kinsella, A., Turner, M. & Barry, S. (1997) Postnatal depression and elation among mothers and their partners: prevalence and predictors. *Br J Psychiatry, 171*, 550-5.

Lawrie, T. A., Hofmeyr, G. J., De Jager, M., Berk, M., Paiker, J. & Viljoen, E. (1998) A double-blind randomised placebo controlled trial of postnatal norethisterone enanthate: the effect on postnatal depression and serum hormones. *Br J Obstet Gynaecol, 105*, 1082-90.

Lommatzsch, M., Hornych, K., Zingler, C., Schuff-Werner, P., Hoppner, J. & Virchow, J. C. (2006) Maternal serum concentrations of BDNF and depression in the perinatal period. *Psychoneuroendocrinology, 31*, 388-94.

Magiakou, M. A., Mastorakos, G., Rabin, D., Dubbert, B., Gold, P. W. & Chrousos, G. P. (1996) Hypothalamic corticotropin-releasing hormone suppression during the postpartum period: implications for the increase in psychiatric manifestations at this time. *J Clin Endocrinol Metab, 81*, 1912-7.

Magiakou, M. A., Mastorakos, G., Webster, E. & Chrousos, G. P. (1997) The hypothalamic-pituitary-adrenal axis and the female reproductive system. *Ann N Y Acad Sci, 816*, 42-56.

Matthey, S., Barnett, B., Howie, P. & Kavanagh, D. J. (2003) Diagnosing postpartum depression in mothers and fathers: whatever happened to anxiety? *Journal of Affective Disorders, 74*, 139-147.

McIvor, R. J., Davies, R. A., Wieck, A., Marks, M. N., Brown, N., Campbell, I. C., Checkley, S. A. & Kumar, R. (1996) The growth hormone response to apomorphine at 4 days postpartum in women with a history of major depression. *J Affect Disord, 40*, 131-6.

Meyer, S. E., Chrousos, G. P. & Gold, P. W. (2001) Major depression and the stress system: a life span perspective. *Dev Psychopathol, 13*, 565-80.

Okano, T. & Nomura, J. (1992) Endocrine study of the maternity blues. *Prog Neuropsychopharmacol Biol Psychiatry, 16*, 921-32.

Owens, P. C., Smith, R., Brinsmead, M. W., Hall, C., Rowley, M., Hurt, D., Lovelock, M., Chan, E. C., Cubis, J. & Lewin, T. (1987) Postnatal disappearance of the pregnancy-associated reduced sensitivity of plasma cortisol to feedback inhibition. *Life Sci, 41*, 1745-50.

Rubinow, D. R., Schmidt, P. J. & Roca, C. A. (1998) Hormone measures in reproductive endocrine-related mood disorders: diagnostic issues. *Psychopharmacol Bull, 34*, 289-90.

Sichel, D. A., Cohen, L. S., Robertson, L. M., Ruttenberg, A. & Rosenbaum, J. F. (1995) Prophylactic estrogen in recurrent postpartum affective disorder. *Biol Psychiatry, 38*, 814-8.

Smith, R. & Thomson, M. (1991) Neuroendocrinology of the hypothalamo-pituitary-adrenal axis in pregnancy and the puerperium. *Baillieres Clin Endocrinol Metab, 5*, 167-86.

Soet, J. E., Brack, G. A. & Diiorio, C. (2003) Prevalence and Predictors of Women's Experience of Psychological Trauma During Childbirth. *Birth, 30*, 36-46.

Stein, G. S. (1980) The pattern of mental change and body weight change in the first post-partum week. *Journal of Psychosomatic Research, 24*, 165-171.

Sugawara, M., Toda, M. A., Shima, S., Mukai, T., Sakakura, K. & Kitamura, T. (1997) Premenstrual mood changes and maternal mental health in pregnancy and the postpartum period. *J Clin Psychol, 53*, 225-32.

Taylor, A., Dore, C. & Glover, V. (1996) Urinary phenylethylamine and cortisol levels in the early puerperium. *J Affect Disord, 37*, 137-42.

Taylor, A., Littlewood, J., Adams, D., Dore, C. & Glover, V. (1994) Serum cortisol levels are related to moods of elation and dysphoria in new mothers. *Psychiatry Res, 54*, 241-7.

Tsigos, C. & Chrousos, G. P. (2002) Hypothalamic-pituitary-adrenal axis, neuroendocrine factors and stress. *J Psychosom Res, 53*, 865-71.

Warner, R., Appleby, L., Whitton, A. & Faragher, B. (1996) Demographic and obstetric risk factors for postnatal psychiatric morbidity. *Br J Psychiatry, 168*, 607-11.

Wieck, A. (1989) Endocrine aspects of postnatal mental disorders. *Baillieres Clin Obstet Gynaecol, 3*, 857-77.

Wieck, A., Kumar, R., Hirst, A. D., Marks, M. N., Campbell, I. C. & Checkley, S. A. (1991) Increased sensitivity of dopamine receptors and recurrence of affective psychosis after childbirth. *Bmj, 303*, 613-6.

In: New Research on Postpartum Depression
Editor: Adrian I. Rosenfield, pp. 85-104
ISBN 1-60021-284-0
© 2007 Nova Science Publishers, Inc.

Chapter VI

MAJOR DEPRESSIVE EPISODE IN POSTPARTUM: A PRELIMINARY PROSPECTIVE 1-YEAR NATURALISTIC FOLLOW-UP

Lluïsa Garcia-Esteve[*], Purificación Navarro-García, Carlos Ascaso Terrén, Jaume Aguado Carné and Anna Torres Giménez

Unit of Perinatal Psychiatry and Gender Research, Consultation-Liaison Psychiatry, Institut Clínic de Neurociències, Hospital Clínic, Barcelona and the Department of Public Health of the University of Barcelona, Barcelona. Institut d'Investigacións Biomèdiques August Pi i Sunyer (IDIBAPS), Spain.

ABSTRACT

Objective

This study examined the 12-month clinical course of major depressive episodes (MDE) in postpartum.

Method

Prospective, naturalistic, longitudinal study with a cohort of 140 women. All subjects were assessed at baseline with the Structured Clinical Interview (SCI) according to DSM-IV criteria for major depressive episode. Follow-up was performed at two, six, twelve, eighteen and twenty-four months using the Longitudinal Interval Follow-up Evaluation (LIFE-UP), to obtain information prospectively on syndrome and overall

---

[*] Correspondence concerning this article should be addressed to Lluïsa Garcia-Esteve, Unitat de Psiquiatria Perinatal i Recerca de Gènere (UPPiRG), Hospital Casa de Maternitat, C/ Sabino de Arana, 1, 08028 Barcelona (España); lesteve@clinic.ub.es.

illness severity and treatment. Kaplan-Meier curves were constructed to assess the likelihood of partial and full remission.

Results

The average follow-up time of the cohort was 41.9 weeks (range: 1-52 weeks). 89.3 % of cohorts completed the 2-month follow-up, while 76.4 % reached the 1-year follow-up. At six-month follow-up, 71,4% (95% CI: 62-78,6%) of women reached, at least, partial remission, while 41,4% (95% CI: 31,8-49,7) achieved full remission. After 1-year follow-up 87,6% (95% CI:79,5-92,5) reached partial and 64% (95% CI: 54-72%) full remission. The median time until partial remission was 16 weeks (95% CI: 13-19 weeks) and 32 weeks (95% CI: 25.5-38.5 weeks) in the case of full remission.

Conclusion

The MDE in postpartum context is not a benign or a transient disorder. Postpartum is not a protective context with respect to prognosis of major depression in mothers. The knowledge that almost a third of mothers with a major depressive episode didn't reach full recovery at 1 year of follow-up may help to refine the guidelines of depression diagnosis and treatment during pregnancy and postpartum.

INTRODUCTION

Maternity has historically been described as a time of emotional well-being, providing protection against psychiatric disorders. However, mental disorders associated with childbearing are a significant Public Health problem. Postpartum major depression is not only associated with morbidity and mortality in affected women, but also with increased morbidity in their children. Pioneer researchers are beginning to provide the prevalence of maternal depression, and they suggest an 8%-13% risk of postnatal depression [1,2]. Our data confirm that 4% met diagnostic DSM-IV criteria for major depression and 6% for minor depression [3]. Only 50% are recognized in clinical practices [4] and less than one third received any type of intervention [5]. There is considerable evidence for the efficacy of therapies for depression. In contrast, treatment during postpartum period is controversial and is based on a limited number of controlled clinical trials [6]. Physicians are reluctant to treat women with drugs during the postpartum for fear of adverse effects on the breastfeeding newborn and because of the high reluctance by mothers. They have the common belief that puerperal episodes are often short-lived, auto limited and may last no more than 3-6 months [7]. However, the duration of postpartum illness appears to be variable and it is not clearly delineated. Two controlled studies found durations of depression to be similar in childbearing and non-childbearing subjects [8,9], but others just the contrary [10]. The course of MDE in non postpartum patients treated with antidepressants has been well established. However, the course in those women who receipt antidepressants during postpartum has not been previously investigated. Long-term patterns of disease in postpartum would be able to gather specific characteristics related to gender and to biological and psychological changes that accompany to childbirth. The few findings of prospective longitudinal studies are heterogeneous and difficult to compare. The samples of depressed mothers were small [11,12,13], based in women with major and minor depression [11-10,7] and among women with specific characteristics, such as first-time mothers, only married or with high cultural level [11-12,7,14-15]. Other postpartum longitudinal broad studies have relied on self-reports of depressive symptoms to diagnose depression at the baseline or for depicting the follow-up course [12,14-15-16] rather than structured clinical interview based on DSM-IV or RDC criteria. In addition, those which used clinical interview rarely specified operational criteria to judge recovery, remission, relapse, or chronicity [13]].

A recent review with twenty-four articles concluded that depressive episodes tend to be longer, more severe and with potential chronicity [17]. This need to be addressed because of the severe long-term consequences for mother and family [18-19]. Postpartum depression substantially decreases maternal functioning [20]. Mothers with a history of postpartum-onset major depression had higher risk of recurrence after the first months of another birth [21], and partners are at significantly higher risk of becoming psychologically distressed themselves [22,12]. Perinatal maternal depression has been associated with lower quality interactions between mothers and their children [23-24], insecurity in attachment relationships [25-26] and increased risk for impaired cognitive [27], and language development [28] as well as psychiatric disturbance among children [29,19]. In addition, missed pediatric appointments and greater use of emergency department services has been observed [30]. The persistence of symptoms during the first postnatal year had special interest because chronicity and severity of postnatal depression are related to the negative effects on the child of the affected mothers [31-32]. Remission of maternal depression was associated with reductions in the children's diagnoses and symptoms, whereas lingering depression may increase the rates of their children's disorders [33].

At present, there are many questions regarding the course of major depression in postpartum. The time for remission and the chronicity must be better explored. How long does an episode of unipolar major depression last after we begin to treat it, in a postpartum context? What's the recovery's rate over time? What is the probability of recurrence after recovery?

The prognosis of a postpartum MDE is an important issue for mothers, familiars and clinicians. It also helps contribute to estimate disease burden and priorizate health care expenditures.

The present paper focuses on the 1-year clinical course of a cohort of women diagnosed in the postpartum as suffering from MDE. The aim of this study was to improve the practical management and health policies of perinatal illness depression.

METHOD

Participants

A total of 140 women were enrolled in a prospective longitudinal naturalistic study, between April 2002 and February 2005. The participants were selected from one center with specific expertise in the treatment of psychiatric illness during pregnancy and postpartum (Unit of Perinatal Psychiatry and Research of Gender, Hospital Clinic of Barcelona). The cohort was recruited from women who were attended at the Obstetric Unit for routine postnatal check-up (six weeks after delivery), and direct referrals from community obstetrical, psychiatric, pediatric and general practices. Participants were included in the study if they 1) had a major depressive episode during postpartum, 2) were less than 6 months postpartum, 3) wished to receive psychological/psychiatric treatment. Patients were excluded if they 1) met Diagnostic and Statistical Manual of Mental Disorders, Fourth Edition (DSM-IV) criteria for one of the following disorders: organic mental disorders; bipolar disorder; schizophrenia; or current psychotic disorder, 2) did not speak Spanish 3) could not read or write 4) had a dead newborn 5) would change residence in the following 2-years.

All patients gave informed consent to participate in the study. The study protocol was approved by the Ethics Committee of Clinical Research of the Clinic Hospital.

Assessment Procedure

Both experienced senior psychiatrist (LG) and trained clinical psychologist (PN) assessed participants at baseline to determine study eligibility. The Structured Clinical Interview (SCID-I/P; [34], depression module, was administered at baseline to confirm a DSM-IV diagnosis of current major depressive episode (MDE). Excellent interrater reliability was achieved for the diagnosis of depression (overall kappa = 0.91) [35]. Melancholia, atypical and psychotic depression were assessed using the DSM-IV criteria. Information regarding variables that might influence the risk of remission was collected including demographic and clinical data. Systematic follow-up was performed by independent interviewers at two, six and twelve months from entry in the study and after any treatment visits using the Longitudinal Interval Follow-up Evaluation (LIFE-UP) [36]. The LIFE assesses psychopathology by employing a six point psychiatric status rating (PSR) scale that is scored on a week-by-week basis at each interview. A PSR score of 6 include full DSM-IV criteria for MDE with either prominent psychotic symptoms or extreme functional impairment. Full symptom criteria without extreme functional impairment, is indicated by a PSR score of 5. A PSR score of 4 indicates less than five major depressive symptoms and moderate functional impairment. A PSR score of 3 include three depressive symptoms for less than 50% of the time. A PSR score of 2 indicates one o two occasional depressive symptoms in mild degree. Lack of symptoms, is indicated by a PSR score of 1.

Table 1. Summary of longitudinal prospective studies relied on diagnosis criteria of postpartum depression.

Authors, year	Sample	Measures	Outcomes	Strengths	Limitations
McMahon C, Barnett B, 2005	100 primiparous mothers, with stable partner and higher education.	CIDI-DSM-IV CES-D>16	60% of those mothers with depressive symptomatology at 4 months had depressive symptoms at 12 months	Major depression at baseline.	No survival analysis Non-representative sample Self-administered measure
Zelkowitz, Milet, 2001	48 mothers	SCID-NP LIFE EPDS	54% psychiatric disorder at 6 months	Standardized diagnostic criteria	Small sample size Heterogeneity of psychiatric diagnoses. No survival analysis. Inexplicit criteria of remission
Areias 1996	54 primiparous mothers	EPDS SADS	49% of those mothers with depressive symptoms at 3 months had depressive disorder at 12 months postpartum		Self-administered measure at baseline
Beeghly M, 2002	106 primiparous mothers.	CES-D>16 Clinical diagnostic interview	One third of the mothers with CES-D >16 at baseline had high scores on CES-D at 3,6, and 12 months of follow up.	Control group	Non-representative sample. No survival analysis Self-administered measure at baseline
Cooper y Murray, 1995	54 primiparous mothers with stable partner	PSI- RDC	70% of mothers with first-onset depression recovered within 1-3 months, 15% within 4-6 months. 38% of mothers with past history of depression recovered within 1-3 months, 30% within 4-6 months.	Antidepressant treatment was controlled	No survival analysis Major and minor postpartum depression included.
Cox JL, Murray, Chapman, 1993	232 childbearing and no childbearing women	EPDS SPI (RDC criteria)	Mean duration of postpartum depression: 36 weeks. Mean duration of non postpartum depression: 50 weeks.	Paired control group	Major and minor depression included. No survival analysis Inexplicit criteria of remission
Campbell SB, Cohn, 1992	70 primiparous mothers with stable partner	SADS RDC			No survival analysis. Non-representative sample
Authors, year	*Sample*	*Measures*	*Outcomes*	*Strengths*	*Limitations*
Cooper PJ, 1988	Community sample of 483 mothers.	PSE-RDC	Only 1/3 of those women with psychiatric disorders at postpartum had psychiatric disorder at 6 months postpartum. The duration minor of 3 months.	Control group. Standardized diagnostic criteria	No survival analysis Heterogeneity of psychiatric diagnoses

Table 1. (Continued)

Authors, year	Sample	Measures	Outcomes	Strengths	Limitations
Kumar and Robson, 1984	114 primiparous mothers. Sample did not receive treatment.	SPI	16% at 3 months 12,5% at 6 months 8,3% at 12 months	Standardized diagnostic criteria Follow up of 4 years	Heterogeneity of psychiatric diagnoses
Watson, 1984	128 randomly selected women	SPI-ICD-9	13% (n=17) psychiatric disorder at pregnancy. 16% (n=20) psychiat-ric disorder at 6 weeks postpartum.	Randomly selected women	Heterogeneity of psychiatric diagnoses

Treatment

The study protocol did not influence the treatment provided by the psychiatrist. However, antidepressant treatment was quantified with the LIFE for each week of the study by means of a 5-point scale "Composite Antidepressant Scale" (CAS). Each point in this scale specified a range of daily doses of imipramine or its equivalent (37). A composite antidepressant score of zero indicated that no antidepressant somatic treatment was provided, a CAS of 1 indicated a daily dose of 1 mg to 149 mg of imipramine or its equivalent, a CAS of 2 indicated daily dose of 150mg to 224 mg of imipramine or its equivalent, a CAS of 3 indicated a daily dose of 225 mg to 299 mg of imipramine or its equivalent, and a composite antidepressant score 4 indicated a daily dose of 300mg or more of imipramine or its equivalent. The addition of lithium, as well as, the combination of two antidepressants increased 1-point the CAS score.

Definitions of Remission and Relapse

As described in the literature (38) (39), recovery from a mood episode or *full remission* required 8 consecutive weeks with a PSR score of 2 or less (minimal or no symptoms). *Partial remission* is defined as a decrease in symptoms with a PSR score of 3 for eight consecutive weeks. The *duration* of an episode was calculated excluding these last 8 weeks in full or partial remission. Patients were considered to be in an episode at baseline if they meet full criteria (PSR=5 or 6) for MDE. Patients who experienced a partial remission were designated as *relapsed* if their PSR score increased to either 5 or 6 (full criteria) for 2 consecutive weeks. *Chronicity* is defined as a PSR score of 6, 5 or 4 during 1-year.

Statistical Analysis

The agreement between inter rater diagnoses was calculated by using the Kappa statistic [35] and the 95% Confidence Interval (95% CI). Fisher's exact tests were used to compare sociodemographic variables between completers and dropouts. The outcome of interest was partial and full remission. The data were censored either by loss to follow-up or end of the assessment period. Survival analysis was used to analyze time until partial or full remission during the period of follow-up (maximum of 52 weeks). The Kaplan-Meier product limit was used to estimate the cumulative probability of remission [40]. A two-tailed alpha of 0.05 was considered statistically significant. Statistical analyses were performed with S-Plus 6.2 and SPSS vs13.0 package software.

RESULTS

A total of 140 postpartum women were entered into the study with a diagnosis of MDE. Of these, 125 (89.3%) were completed the two months, 115 (82.1%) the six months and 107 (76.4%) the one year follow up. The average follow up time of all women was 41.9 weeks (range 1-52; SD= 18.2). Of the 140 women who were followed up across the study, 25 were lost to follow-up and 8 choose to discontinue participation in the study. We found differences between women who completed the 1-year follow-up (n=107) and women who dropped out (n=33) in financial difficulties ($p<0,01$, Fisher's exact test), maternal employment status ($p<0,05$, Fisher's exact test) and pregnancy planning ($p<0,01$, Fisher's exact test). Women who dropped out from the study had more often financial difficulties (51.5% vs. 21.5%), were more often unemployed during the pregnancy (27.3% vs. 11.2%), and had more often unplanned pregnancy (48.5% vs. 31.7%) than mothers who completed the follow up.

Sociodemographic and Clinical Characteristics

Table 2 illustrates the demographic characteristics of all participants. Overall, the mean age of participants was 32.2 years (SD=4.77). Most women were Spanish (87.1%). Approximately 60% of participants reported completing a secondary or superior level of the education and were first-time mothers, and 99% had a stable partner. Seventy per cent had not financial difficulties, and 85% were employed during the pregnancy. Approximately one third had an unplanned pregnancy and 49% breastfed their children at onset of follow up.

Clinical characteristics of the sample are presented in table 3. The large majority (76.4%) of the cohort was characterized by a index major depressive episode with postpartum-onset. 28% met DSM-IV criteria for melancholia, and 3% met DSM-IV criteria for psychotic major depressive episode. Half of them had first-onset major depressive episode, and 42% had first-degree familial history of affective disorders. In all, 13.6% did not receive antidepressant treatment during the study.

Table 2. Demographic Characteristics of Postpartum Women with a Major Depressive Episode.

Variables	All (N=140)	
	N	%
Country of birth		
Spain	122	87.1
Other countries	18	12.9
Aged		
≤18	1	0.7
19-34	100	71.4
≥35	39	27.9
Level of education		
None	9	6.4
Primary	43	30.7
Secondary	51	36.4
Superior	37	26.4
Current marital status		
Live in partner or married	138	98.6
Single	2	1.4
Parity		
Primiparous	85	60.7
Secundiparous	45	32.1
Multiparous	10	7.1
Financial difficulties		
No	100	71.4
Yes	40	28.6
Pregnancy employment status		
Employed	119	85
Unemployed	21	15
Breast-feeding status at baseline		
Yes	68	48.6
No	72	51.4
Pregnancy planning		
Yes	90	64.3
No, but accepted	40	28.6
No, it was an accident	10	7.1

Table 3. Clinical Characteristics of Postpartum Women with a Major Depressive Episode (n=140)

Variables	Participants 1ª visita (n=140)	
	N	%
Index episode		
Onset of current episode		
Before pregnancy	18	12.9
During pregnancy	15	10.7
After delivery	107	76.4
DSM-IV major depressive episode subtypes		
Melancholia	39	27.9
Atypical depression	36	25.7
Psicotic depression	4	2.9
Prior treated depressive episode		
No	77	55.0
Yes	63	45.0
HDRS* at baseline	140	23.36 (SD=6.40)
Antidepressant treatment across the study		
No	23	16.4
Yes	117	83.6
Personal psychiatric history		
History of hospitalisations	5	3.6
History of suicide attempts	11	7.9
History of lifetime affective disorders (treated or not)	89	63.6
No. Of prior postpartum depressive episodes		
Never pregnant	85	60.7
None	40	28.6
≥1	15	10.7
Family psychiatric history		
First-degree family history of psychiatric illness	82	58.6
First-degree family history of depression	59	42.1
First-degree family history of suicide	8	5.7

*Hamilton Depression Rating Scale

Partial Remission

We recorded at least partial remission in 103 (73.6%) of our cohort. Thirteen women (9.3%) never satisfied the partial remission criteria for the 52 weeks of follow-up. The follow-up was incomplete in 24 (17.1%) women without ever attaining partial remission.

Figure 1 shows the cumulative probability of remaining in the index major depressive episode for the total cohort: 33.5% (95% CI: 25-41%) recovered within 2 months, 71.4% (95% CI: 62-78.6%) recovered within 6 months and 87.6% (95% CI: 79.5-92.5%) recovered at 12 months of follow-up. At 1 year follow-up 12,6% (95% CI: 7.2-18.7) did not reach partial remission. The median duration of an episode after entry into the study was 16 weeks (95% CI: 13-19 weeks). The mean duration with the upper limit of 52 weeks was 20.2 weeks (95% CI: 17.4-23.1). We can observe that major incidence of partial remissions occurs during the first semester after entry in the study.

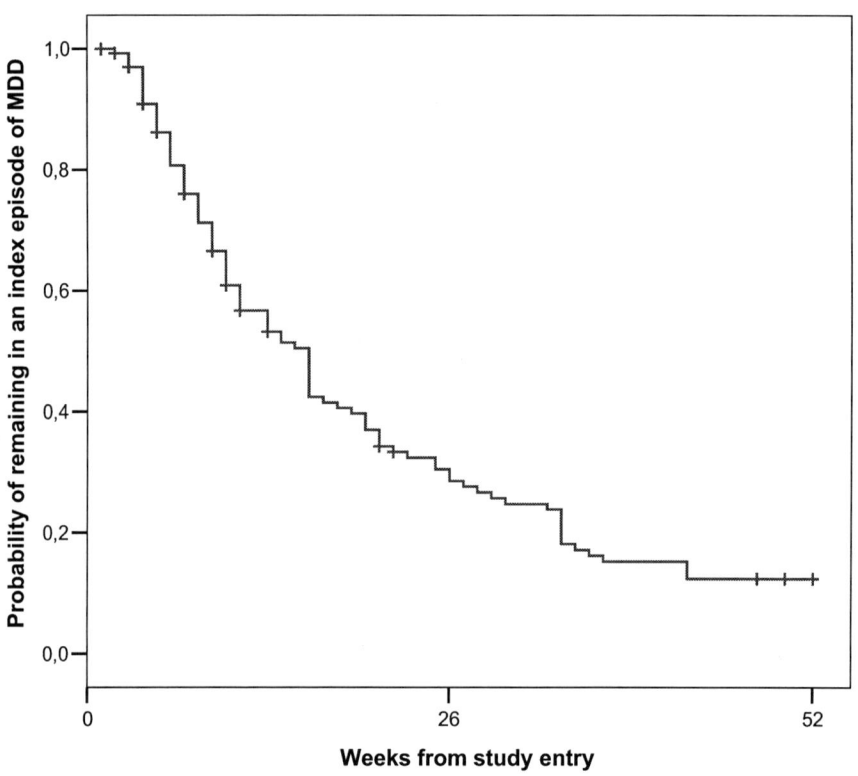

Figure 1. Time to at least partial remission and probabilty of remaining in the index episode after entry in the study for the 140 postpartum women with DSM-IV Major Depressive Episode (MDE).

Recovery or Full Remission

We recorded full remission in 74 (53%) of our cohort. Forty women (28.6%) never satisfied the full remission criteria for the 52 weeks of follow-up. The follow-up was incomplete in 26 (18.5%) women without ever attaining full remission. Figure 2 shows the cumulative probability of remaining in the index major depressive episode for the total cohort: 10.2% (95% CI: 5-15.2%) full recovered within 2 months, 41.4% (95% CI: 31.8-49.7%) recovered within 6 months and 64% (95% CI: 54-72%) recovered at 12 months of follow-up. At 1 year follow-up 36% (95% CI: 27.8-44.2) did not reach full remission Five women (4.7%; 95% CI:1.5-10.6) were still in the index episode at 12 months of follow-up.

The median duration of an episode after entry into the study was 32 weeks (95% CI: 25.5-38.5 weeks). The mean duration with the upper limit of 52 weeks was 33.1 weeks (95% CI: 30-36). We can observe that during the two first months after entry in the study the incidence per month of full remissions is low, but from this point it increases being constant until 10-months follow-up, then it level-off and this fact can be interpreted as a first attainment of a first remission threshold.

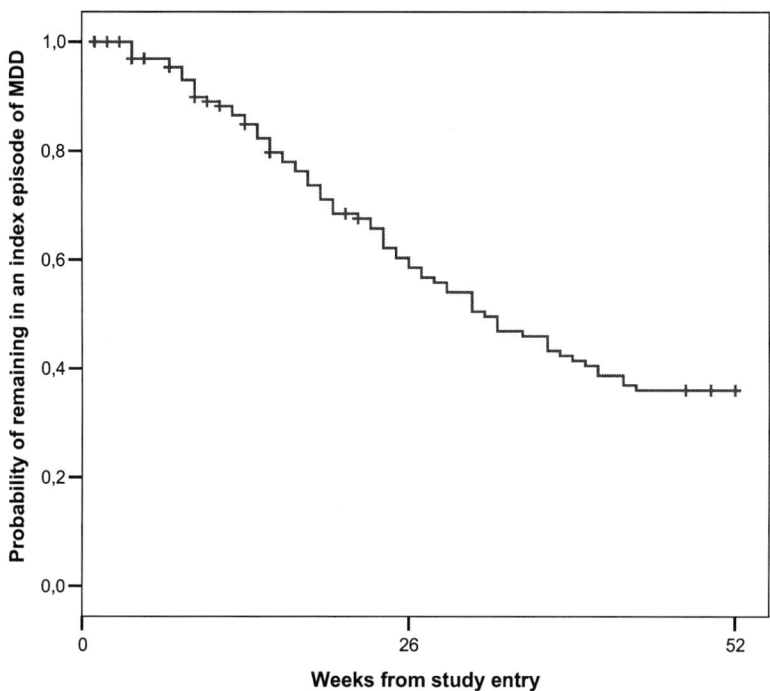

Figure 2. Time to full remission and probabilty of remaining in the index episode after entry in the study for the 140 postpartum women with DSM-IV Major Depressive Episode (MDE).

Relapse Rate

Among the 103 women that previously reached at least partial remission, 8 (7.8%) experienced a relapse within the 1-year follow-up, 86 (83.5%) never experienced a relapse during the 1-year follow-up and 9 (8.7%) women were lost to follow-up. At 2-months from partial remission any women presented a relapse, at 6-months 5 (5.6%) (95% CI: 0.7-10.2) women had been a relapse, and at 12-moths of follow-up 8 (10.4%) (95% CI:3-17.1) women relapsed.

Symptoms Level During the Episode (PSR)

Figure 3 shows the symptoms level in function of the time for still sick patients. A patient that begin its recovery (got a PSR score of 1 or 2 during 8 consecutive weeks), in a determinate week is censored from analysis in the following weeks. Symptoms level during the index episode begins with a mean PSR of 5, because one of the inclusion criteria was meeting MDE DSM-IV criteria. PSR decreases just fewer than 4, at the end of the 2-month follow-up, ranging in a narrow interval of 3-3.5 during the remaining year of follow-up.

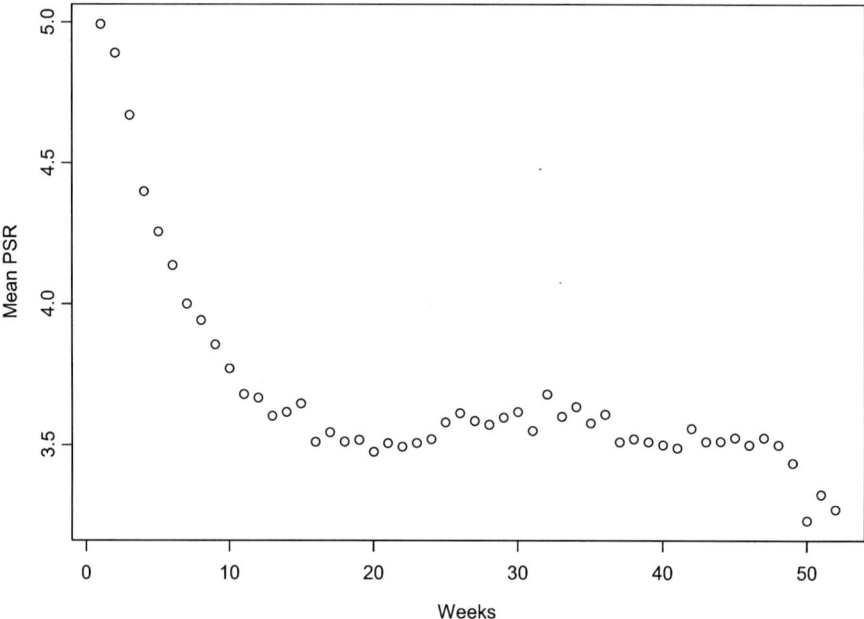

Figure 3. Symptoms level by 1-year follow-up for still sick patients.

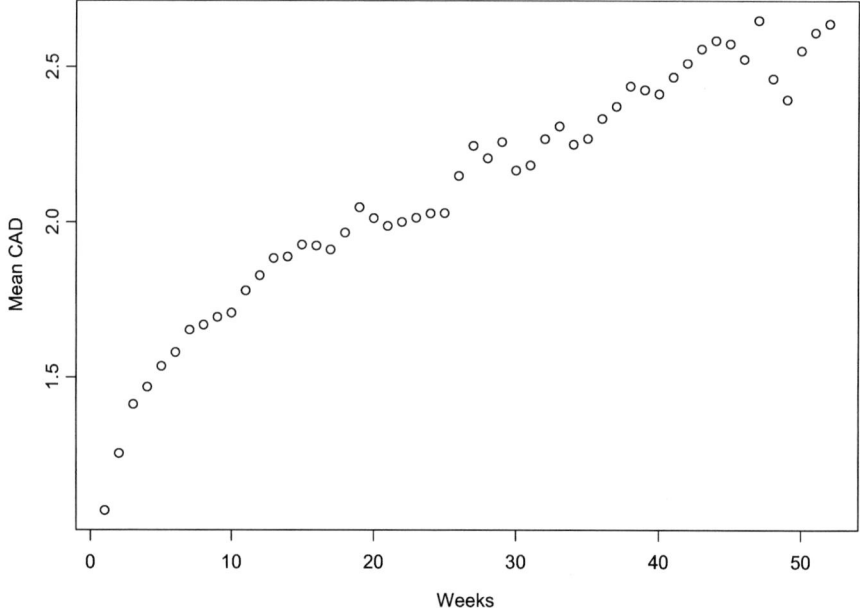

Figure 4. Mean antidepressant CAD sco re by 1-year follow-up for the still sick patients.

Level of Antidepressant Treatment (CAD)

Received treatment during the index episode was resumed by mean of CAD score (see Figure 4). We calculated the mean CAD score for each week for all the still sick and active in the study patients. As we can observe in the CAD figure, at the beginning of the study mean treatment is 1, because there are few subjects under treatment or beginning it, despite of meet complete criteria for depression. Later on, we observe a gradual increase of antidepressant treatment intensity until to reach therapeutic doses in 20 weeks. From the week 20 and until the end of follow-up treatment doses were increased in a continuous fashion until achieve a CAD score of 2.5.

DISCUSSION

To our knowledge, this is the first prospective longitudinal, naturalistic follow-up study that describes the course of major depressive episode in a wide cohort of postpartum women who were referred to a Perinatal Unit of Psychiatry to received psychiatric management. It extends our previous first published data about postpartum depression [3,41-42] and provides additional data on its recovery and course outcome. The general findings highlight that major depressive episode in postpartum is not a short and benign disorder, even under treatment. We find that over the 1-year follow-up, only 64% of postpartum outpatient women recovered from their index episode and 88% achieved partial remission. Furthermore, there were 36% who need more time to reached full remission, 12% of women continued to report elevated symptoms, 5% remained in the index episode and 10% relapsed after partial remission. The median time from entry into the study until full remission was 32 weeks and 16 weeks until partial remission.

The temporal evolution for partial and full remission was different across the follow-up. The probability of full remission during the first two months was smaller than for partial remission. At 2-months, only 10% reached a full remission, while one third decreased until partial remission. At 3-months, there was a rapid incidence of full remission, it kept constant until 10-months and then leveled off. Partial remission presented a rapid and constant incidence until 6-months and then often leveled off. Monthly rates of either partial or full remission declined abruptly for the remaining two months of the 1-year follow-up. It suggests that the women who did not reach full remission stand for a treatment resistant group. The difference in temporal evolution for both type of remissions supports the hypothesis that partial remission is more frequent during the onset of follow-up and may could be present in the absence of treatment. In contrast, full remission was related with the onset of treatment and this only could be present if previously has been reached therapeutically dose. Thus, the rate of full remission was depending on the frame time when treatment achieved therapeutically dose. The observed delay in the rates of full remission during the first months could be attributed to the reluctance's mothers to use psychiatric medications after delivery, especially among lactating women. All women received information about the risk of adverse effects related to medication exposure, the benefit of breastfeed, and the adverse effects of untreated maternal depression. Moreover, pharmacological treatment and breastfeeding with pediatric controls, were recommended. When mother's agreed, antidepressant treatment was introduced gradually, reaching therapeutically dose at 4-months follow-up.

In general, our results indicated lower recovery's rate at 6 and 12 months follow-up than previous longitudinal studies in postpartum and non postpartum samples. Prospective studies in postpartum samples, found that two third recovered at 6 months postpartum, [11,43], and from 76% to 92.5% at 1-year postpartum [7,11]. In non-postpartum samples, severity and length of depressive symptoms were associated with recovery's delay [39,44]. Our sample is based only on women with a MDE, with moderate to severe symptoms, 28% melancholic and 3% psychotic symptoms. We do not know exactly the time from onset of the MDE, except that 76% had a postpartum onset, 11% during pregnancy and 13 % before pregnancy. The inclusion of a long lasting subgroup may explain a longer recovery. It would be necessary future analyses related with the onset of the episode. However, other factors belonging to depressive spectrum could take into account it. We would like to point out that a half of mothers had a previous treated episode, and first-degree family history of depression. One third of non first–mothers had previous postpartum depression episodes. Moreover, one third of the total sample had an unplanned pregnancy.

In contrast, our recovery's rate is two-fold higher than 20% reported by Zelkowitz and Millet (2001) [13] at 6 months, in the only postpartum study that used the LIFE. However, this study was restricted to a small sample of non treated women.

The studies in non pospartum MDE using the same defined criteria about recovery, showed a better cumulative probability of full remission ranging from 50% to 77% at 6 months [39,45-46], and from 70% to 85% at 1-year [39,46]. The median time for full remission was 6 months. However, in our cohort, the median time to achieve full remission was 8 months, and more than 4 months for partial remission, after it came under medical management. Most of these studies were carried out in male and female inpatients who received antidepressant treatment prior or just at baseline [39,45,46,47].

Both of our rates of relapse and chronicity are smaller than in other studies but it could be necessary continuing the follow up study before conclusion

Our data indicated that MDE in postpartum from a longitudinal perspective, is a serious illnesses. It has a potential long-lasting course that could be related to gender differences during childbearing years. This disorder can be resistant or respond with a long delay to conventional psychiatric treatment methods. Longitudinal course of depression may differ between men and women and the average length of episode is longer in women [48,49]. Moreover, in postpartum context there could be many others reasons to explain the longest course: 1) The delay in the onset of treatment relating to breastfeed, 2) The involvement of reproductive hormones, thyroid and hypothalamus-pituitary-ovarian axis in postpartum depression 3) The prolonged postpartum estradiol's deficiency may produce a resistance in the treatment antidepressant response [50], 4) The frequents anxiety and obsessive symptoms and comorbid disorders in this population do depression more resistant to recovery, 5) In postpartum mothers, perceived stress and resources to cope with demands are affected by the physical state (i.e., anemia, tiredness, sleep disturbances). At the same time, family care giving are superimposed to the constant attention to the newborn, and mothers do not follow preventive health behaviors, such as rest and exercise, nor do they seek social support, 6)

Finally, in our study 85% are working's mothers and they must to return to work at five months postpartum. This made mothers in difficulty to combine work and motherhood.

In conclusion, postpartum is not a protective context to prognosis of MDE. Our data suggest that mothers with a diagnostic of a MDE in the postpartum, even under by treatment, are likely to remain with depressive symptoms at six months, and a subgroup more than 12 months. Our findings have some clinical implications. On the other hand, prompt detection of maternal depression and early interventions are important, because the degree of risk to children appears related to the duration of the mother's depression [51] and can significantly reduce adverse consequences to both mothers and children. On the other hand, many women who decide to discontinue antidepressant treatment to conceive or during pregnancy will experience recurrent depressive episode before [52] or after delivery. The knowledge that one third of depressive mothers didn't reached full remission at 1 year, may help clinicians and women to refine the risk-benefit decision for treatment during pregnancy and postpartum. Women should be aware of the risk of suffering from long lasting depression during one year after delivery if they experience a major depressive episode in postpartum.

Strengths

This study has a number of strengths. First, it was designed from the perspective of what clinicians need to know about typical postpartum cases of major depression in public practice. Second, we performed prospective, serial assessment using standardized instruments and multiple regular-interval week by week follow-up during a period of 1-year. Because estimates of episode length may show-up to seven fold variation, depending on the definition of recovery [53], we applied predefined operational criteria, in accordance with the NIMH criteria to determine partial and full remission, relapse and chronicity. This study was less subject to referral filter bias than studies conducted on in-patients.

Limitation

Although this study is a unique contribution to the literature on postpartum naturalistic course of major depressive episode in outpatients, several limitations deserve some comments. As with any prospective interview study in which subjects are asked to recall mood symptoms since the most recent assessment, the information gathered is subject to multiple sources of inerrability. Our efforts to maximize the accuracy of the information obtained included attempts to interview subjects for follow-up after any visit of treatment with an independent interviewer. Because subjects were recruited from clinical outpatient settings, the results of this study cannot be generalized to other postpartum populations. Decisions about the onset of treatment were made by mothers after they received the information about risk/benefit. Psychopharmacological treatment was recorded but uncontrolled and psychotherapy treatment was not assessed. Another limitation was that 23.6% of women drop out prior to finish the study. The high proportion of low-income mothers among drop out women is consistent with previous reports that depressed low-income women do not use community care available to them, even if it is free [54]. Subjects were recruited in different time of onset of their index episode. Finally, we did not examine the predictive course's factors of MDE in postpartum but this should be the purpose for future research.

CONCLUSION

Maternity is not a protective factor for severity and prognosis of major depression in women. In most cases, MDE in postpartum is a seriously impairing episodic disease.

The median time to recovery of a MDE that began or relapsed in postpartum context was 33 weeks, after it came under psychiatric management.

The recovery's rate was smaller than we expected. 10% of the cohort reached full remission by 2 months, 41% by 6 months, and 64% by 12 months.

After 1-year follow up, 12% did not achieve partial remission and 5% remained in the index episode.

Our findings highlight the long lasting evolution of MDE in postpartum context, and may help to refine depression treatment guidelines during pregnancy and postpartum.

ACKNOWLEDGMENTS

Supported by grant 011910 from La Fundació la Marató TV3

REFERENCES

[1]   Gavin NI, Gaynes BN, Lohr KN, Meltzer-Brody S, Gartlehner G, Swinson T. Perinatal depression: a systematic review of prevalence and incidence. *Obstet Gynecol* 2005;106:1071-83.

[2]   O'Hara MW, Swain AM. Rates and risk of postpartum depression: A meta-Analysis. *Int Rev Psychiatry* 1996;8:37-54.

[3]   Ascaso TC, Garcia EL, Navarro P, Aguado J, Ojuel J, Tarragona MJ. [Prevalence of postpartum depression in Spanish mothers: comparison of estimation by mean of the structured clinical interview for DSM-IV with the Edinburgh Postnatal Depression Scale]. *Med Clin (Barc)* 2003;120(9):326-9.

[4]   Yonkers KA, Chantilis SJ. Recognition of depression in obstetric/gynecology practices. *Am J Obstet Gynecol* 1995;173(2):632-8.

[5]   Oates MR, Cox JL, Neema S, Asten P, Glangeaud-Freudenthal N, Figueiredo B, et al. Postnatal depression across countries and cultures: a qualitative study. *Br J Psychiatry Suppl* 2004;46:s10-s16.

[6]   Dennis CL. Psychosocial and psychological interventions for prevention of postnatal depression: systematic review. *BMJ* 2005;331(7507):15.

[7] Cooper PJ, Murray L. Course and recurrence of postnatal depression. Evidence for the specificity of the diagnostic concept. *Br J Psychiatry* 1995;166(2):191-5.

[8] O'Hara MW, Zekoski EM, Philipps LH, Wright EJ. Controlled prospective study of postpartum mood disorders: comparison of childbearing and nonchildbearing women. *J Abnorm Psychol* 1990;99(1):3-15.

[9] Whiffen VE, Gotlib IH. Comparison of postpartum and nonpostpartum depression: clinical presentation, psychiatric history, and psychosocial functioning. *J Consult Clin Psychol* 1993;61(3):485-94.

[10] Cox JL, Murray D, Chapman G. A controlled study of the onset, duration and prevalence of postnatal depression. *Br J Psychiatry* 1993;163:27-31.

[11] Campbell SB, Cohn JF, Flanagan C, Popper S, Meyers T. Course and correlates of postpartum depression during the transition to parenthood. *Dev Psychopatholol* 1992;4:29-47.

[12] Areias ME, Kumar R, Barros H, Figueiredo E. Comparative incidence of depression in women and men, during pregnancy and after childbirth. Validation of the Edinburgh Postnatal Depression Scale in Portuguese mothers. *Br J Psychiatry* 1996;169(1):30-5.

[13] Zelkowitz P, Milet TH. The course of postpartum psychiatric disorders in women and their partners. *J Nerv Ment Dis* 2001;189(9):575-82.

[14] Beeghly M, Weinberg MK, Olson KL, Kernan H, Riley J, Tronick EZ. Stability and change in level of maternal depressive symptomatology during the first postpartum year. *J Affect Disord* 2002;71(1-3):169-80.

[15] McMahon C, Barnett B, Kowalenko N, Tennant C. Psychological factors associated with persistent postnatal depression: past and current relationships, defence styles and the mediating role of insecure attachment style. *J Affect Disord* 2005;84(1):15-24.

[16] Horowitz JA, Goodman J. A longitudinal study of maternal postpartum depression symptoms. *Res Theory Nurs Pract* 2004;18(2-3):149-63.

[17] Goodman JH. Postpartum depression beyond the early postpartum period. *J Obstet Gynecol Neonatal Nurs* 2004;33(4):410-20.

[18] Beck CT. The effects of postpartum depression on child development: a meta-analysis. *Arch Psychiatr Nurs* 1998;12(1):12-20.

[19] Philipps LH, O'Hara MW. Prospective study of postpartum depression: 4 1/2-year follow-up of women and children. *J Abnorm Psychol* 1991;100(2):151-5.

[20] Weinberg MK, Tronick EZ, Beeghly M, Olson KL, Kernan H, Riley JM. Subsyndromal depressive symptoms and major depression in postpartum women. *Am J Orthopsychiatry* 2001;71(1):87-97.

[21] Wisner KL, Perel JM, Peindl KS, Hanusa BH. Timing of depression recurrence in the first year after birth. *J Affect Disord* 2004;78(3):249-52.

[22] Ballard CG, Davis R, Cullen PC, Mohan RN, Dean C. Prevalence of postnatal psychiatric morbidity in mothers and fathers. *Br J Psychiatry* 1994;164(6):782-8.

[23] Stein A, Gath DH, Bucher J, Bond A, Day A, Cooper PJ. The relationship between post-natal depression and mother-child interaction. *Br J Psychiatry* 1991 Jan;158:46-52.

[24] Reck C, Hunt A, Fuchs T, Weiss R, Noon A, Moehler E, et al. Interactive regulation of affect in postpartum depressed mothers and their infants: an overview. *Psychopathology* 2004;37(6):272-80.
[25] Cicchetti D, Rogosch FA, Toth SL. Maternal depressive disorder and contextual risk: contributions to the development of attachment insecurity and behavior problems in toddlerhood. *Dev Psychopathol* 1998;10(2):283-300.
[26] Marmorstein NR, Malone SM, Iacono WG. Psychiatric disorders among offspring of depressed mothers: associations with paternal psychopathology. *Am J Psychiatry* 2004;161(9):1588-94.
[27] Murray L. The impact of postnatal depression on infant development. *J Child Psychol Psychiatry* 1992;33(3):543-61.
[28] Field T. Alleviating stress in newborn infants in the intensive care unit. *Clin Perinatol* 1990;17(1):1-9.
[29] Murray L, Stein A. The effects of postnatal depression on the infant. *Baillieres Clin Obstet Gynaecol* 1989;3(4):921-33.
[30] Flynn HA, Davis M, Marcus SM, Cunningham R, Blow FC. Rates of maternal depression in pediatric emergency department and relationship to child service utilization. *Gen Hosp Psychiatry* 2004;26(4):316-22.
[31] Brennan PA, Hammen C, Andersen MJ, Bor W, Najman JM, Williams GM. Chronicity, severity, and timing of maternal depressive symptoms: relationships with child outcomes at age 5. *Dev Psychol* 2000;36(6):759-66.
[32] Campbell SB. Behavior problems in preschool children: a review of recent research. *J Child Psychol Psychiatry* 1995;36(1):113-49.
[33] Weissman MM, Pilowsky DJ, Wickramaratne PJ, Talati A, Wisniewski SR, Fava M, et al. Remissions in maternal depression and child psychopathology: a STAR*D-child report. *JAMA* 2006;295(12):1389-98.
[34] First MB, Spitzer R.L., Gibbon M., Williams J.B.W. Stuctured Clinical Interview for DSM-IV Axis I Disorders-Patient Edition (SCID-I/P, Version 2.0). New York: NY State Psychiatric Instute, Biometrics Research Dept; 1995.
[35] Cohen J. A coefficient of agreement for nominal scales. *Educationaal and psychol Measurement* 1960;20:37-46.
[36] Keller MB, Lavori PW, Friedman B, Nielsen E, Endicott J, Donald-Scott P, et al. The Longitudinal Interval Follow-up Evaluation. A comprehensive method for assessing outcome in prospective longitudinal studies. *Arch Gen Psychiatry* 1987;44(6):540-8.
[37] Keller MB. Undertreatment of major depression. Psychopharmacol Bull 1988;24(1):75-80.
[38] Frank E, Prien RF, Jarrett RB, Keller MB, Kupfer DJ, Lavori PW, et al. Conceptualization and rationale for consensus definitions of terms in major depressive disorder. Remission, recovery, relapse, and recurrence. *Arch Gen Psychiatry* 1991;48(9):851-5.
[39] Keller MB, Lavori PW, Mueller TI, Endicott J, Coryell W, Hirschfeld RM, et al. Time to recovery, chronicity, and levels of psychopathology in major depression. A 5-year prospective follow-up of 431 subjects. *Arch Gen Psychiatry* 1992;49(10):809-16.

[40] Kaplan EL, Meier P. Non-parametric estimations from incomplete observations. *J Am Stat Assoc* 1958;53:457-81.

[41] Garcia-Esteve L, Ascaso C, Ojuel J, Navarro P. Validation of the Edinburgh Postnatal Depression Scale (EPDS) in Spanish mothers. *J Affect Disord* 2003;75(1):71-6.

[42] Garcia-Esteve L, Torres A, Navarro P, Aguado J, Ascaso C. Maternidad no planificada y psicomorbilidad: un riesgo evitable. *Rev psiquiatria Fac Med Barna* 2005;32(3):111-8.

[43] Cooper PJ, Campbell EA, Day A, Kennerley H, Bond A. Non-psychotic psychiatric disorder after childbirth. A prospective study of prevalence, incidence, course and nature. *Br J Psychiatry* 1988;152:799-806.

[44] Ramana R, Paykel ES, Cooper Z, Hayhurst H, Saxty M, Surtees PG. Remission and relapse in major depression: a two-year prospective follow-up study. *Psychol Med* 1995;25(6):1161-70.

[45] Pintor L, Torres X, Navarro V, Gasto C. [Major depressive episode: a study of remission and relapses]. *Med Clin (Barc)* 2002;118(2):41-6.

[46] Furukawa TAFTFKTAKTFTKATK. Time to recovery of an inception cohort with hitherto untreated unipolar major depressive episodes. *Br J Psychiatry* 2000;177:331-5.

[47] Angst J, Preisig M. Outcome of a clinical cohort of unipolar, bipolar and schizoaffective patients. Results of a prospective study from 1959 to 1985. *Schweiz Arch Neurol Psychiatr* 1995;146(1):17-23.

[48] Paykel ES, Ramana R, Cooper Z, Hayhurst H, Kerr J, Barocka A. Residual symptoms after partial remission: an important outcome in depression. *Psychol Med* 1995;25(6):1171-80.

[49] Ernst C, Angst J. The Zurich Study. XII. Sex differences in depression. Evidence from longitudinal epidemiological data. *Eur Arch Psychiatry Clin Neurosci* 1992;241(4):222-30.

[50] Ahokas A, Kaukoranta J, Wahlbeck K, Aito M. Estrogen deficiency in severe postpartum depression: successful treatment with sublingual physiologic 17beta-estradiol: a preliminary study. *J Clin Psychiatry* 2001;62(5):332-6.

[51] Field T, Estroff DB, Yando R, del VC, Malphurs J, Hart S. "Depressed" mothers' perceptions of infant vulnerability are related to later development. *Child Psychiatry Hum Dev* 1996;27(1):43-53.

[52] Cohen LS, Altshuler LL, Harlow BL, Nonacs R, Newport DJ, Viguera AC, et al. Relapse of major depression during pregnancy in women who maintain or discontinue antidepressant treatment. *JAMA* 2006;295(5):499-507.

[53] Philipp M, Fickinger MP. The definition of remission and its impact on the length of a depressive episode. *Arch Gen Psychiatry* 1993;50(5):407-8.

[54] Verdeli H, Ferro T, Wickramaratne P, Greenwald S, Blanco C, Weissman MM. Treatment of depressed mothers of depressed children: pilot study of feasibility. *Depress Anxiety* 2004;19(1):51-8.

Chapter VII

POSTPARTUM DEPRESSION AND CHILDREARING STYLE ON CHILD DEVELOPMENT

Alfonso Pedrós-Roselló[*]

Lluís Alcanyís Hospital, Xátiva 46800, Valencia, Spain.

ABSTRACT

Introduction

There are studies which describe association between postpartum depression and child development, but they lack methodological uniformity. In this work we study the influence of the postpartum depression on child development during the first twenty-eight months of life. We study also the childrearing style of the mother, as the possible mediator of the relationship between postpartum depression and child development.

Methods

It is a longitudinal and prospective study including 205 primipara mothers and their children. The definitive sample includes 23 depressed women and 37 women belonging to the control group. The assessments were carried out independently and blindly at the third day after the delivery and at the 1st, 3rd, 6th, 12th and 28th months. The clinical assessment of the mother was made through a clinical interview, the Present State Examination, and a scale of social adaptation. The childrearing received by the mother during her childhood and adolescence was assessed through the Perceived Childrearing Assesment Questionaire, based on the Parental Bonding Instrument developed by Parker. The childrearing received by the children was studied through an instrument based on the

---

[*] Correspondence concerning this article should be addressed to

direct observation at home of the interaction between the mother and her child at varied ecologic circumstances. Two aspects of the interaction mother-child were assessed: 'affection' and 'care'. The development of the children was assessed using Barley scales of infant development. It was also studied the social development using Stein scale.

Results

A 13.5 % of the women studied have postpartum depression. There are not significant differences regarding perceived childrearing between depressed women and the control group. However, studying the childrearing style of depressed women we observe they bring up their children with a lower level of affection and care than the control group. The length of the depression was determinant in maintaining this lower level of affection and care. During the first year of life, the childrearing style low in affection is associated negatively with the cognitive and social development of the children. At the 28th month the association of a long-course depression and the childrearing style low in affection, during the first year of life, has a negative effect on the cognitive development of the children.

Conclusion

Women with postpartum depression bring up their children with a lower level of affection and care. During the period under study the variable with more weight on the development of the children was a childrearing style low in affection.

Keywords: Postpartum depression, childrearing, mother-child relationship, child development

INTRODUCTION

The relationship established by the mother with her child, and which comes determined by her diverse individual features, defines the model or style of childrearing. Among these features it must be emphasised the postpartum depression which, as it has been demonstrated, determines an altered development in the child. The prevalence of the depression in the postpartum period is situated among the 11-20%, depending on the diagnostic criteria used [1-5].

All the studies suggest that the maternal depressive conduct may be transmitted to the child at the earliest months of life, but the way in which it causes these alterations is still unknown. Diverse possibilities or theoretical expositions are handled: interactions mother-child, imitation by the babies of the maternal conduct or, simply, lack of stimulus [6,7]. The relationship of the depressed mother with her child has been defined as "negative", emphasising the rejection, the hostility, the criticism and emotional indifference [8-10]. The mother reports adverse self-perceptions of her maternal capacities [11], and some alterations have been observed in her interaction with the child [12]. The mother shows frequent difficulties in the management and care of the child, which is reflected in an anomalous childrearing [13,14].

When the mother focuses her attention on the child or on her maternal task, the relationship mother-child, as well as the development of the infant can be negatively affected [15-17]. It seems to exist a relation between the postpartum depression and a delay in the cognitive development of the child, already appreciated in the first months, as well as in subsequent periods [18-21]. The influence of the postpartum depression on the psychomotor development of the child is not confirmed enough [19]. On the other hand, the children of mothers with postpartum depression show a lower social development, normally established at the eighteen months [10,21].

The interest of these investigations goes towards the prevention and treatment of the postpartum depression, carried out by diverse studies directed to the establishment of specific programs in this fundamental phase of the relationship mother-child [22-24].

Revising this subject is observed that: 1º the investigations are limited; 2º little uniformity exists in the design and method; 3º it is usually valued only the existence or not of postpartum depression; 4º only partial aspects of the development of the child are studied and 5º other variables are not studied, such as the style of childrearing.

This study stems from the necessity to deepen in these features of the investigation. The hypothesis of this work are:

1. The postpartum depression of primipara mothers influences in a negative way on the cognitive, psychomotor and social development of the children during the first 28 months of life.
2. The process by which this influence is exercised through the style of childrearing practised by the mother on her child during the first 12 months of life and this is distinguished for a lower "affection" and "care".

METHODS

Material

It is a longitudinal and prospective follow up study. It is carried out on the women who give birth in the Maternity Unit of the Hospital Clínico Universitario de Valencia. The inclusion criteria are: 1. to give birth in the Hospital Clínico Universitario de Valencia and 2. to be primipara mother. The informed consent was requested to the participating women. The criteria of exclusion are: 1. the current presence of psychiatric symtomatology in the mother, with the purpose to exclude those women who presented depressive clinic during the pregnancy, as well as the immediate start after the birth and that would be diagnosed as maternity blue 2. incapacity for the comprehension of the tests and interviews and 3. presence of syndrome of Down or serious malformations in the child.

Variables Studied

The variables studied are:

1. Sociodemographical variables (age, marital status, level of education, work situation before the childbirth and economic incomes of the family).
2. Duration of the postpartum depression, as independent variable.
3. Style of childrearing carried out by the mother ("affection" and "care"), as a mediator variable. At the same time it is studied the style of childrearing perceived by the mother during her infancy and adolescence as a possible distinguishing factor between depressed and not depressed mothers and her posterior interaction with the child.
4. Development of the child (cognitive, psychomotor and social), as dependent variables. These are the fundamental variables of the investigation. Likewise, other variables that could have an effect on the development of the child have been considered:
5. Variables or factors of confusion; these are, the number of perinatal complications experienced by the child, the age of the mother, her level of education, and the economic incomes of the family.

Instruments Used

Postpartum depression. The appraisal is carried out by means of a clinical interview, the Present State Examination (PSE) [25] and a scale of Social Adaptation [26]. This last one consists in a non-structured open interview, with an analogical visual scale of five steps.

Style of childrearing of the mother. A scale is used for the appraisal of the style of childrearing (scale of Negative Maternal Conduct), designed by the authors for the present study. It is an instrument based on the method of the direct observation of the interaction mother-child at home, during different ecological situations such as, the diet, the change of nappies and the bath of the child. Its theoretical base is found in the conception of the style of childrearing developed by Parker [27]. Two aspects or parameters are evaluated. These are "affection" and "care". Thus, two childrearing style scores are obtained, known as style of childrearing low in affection (SRLA) and style of childrearing low in care (SRLC). All these observations are carried for a blind interviewer to the clinical situation of the mother. The scores of the style of childrearing are obtained by the sum of the scores of the appraisals during the analysed period of time. The internal consistence of the instrument is alpha = 0.83, the correlation test-retest = 0.82 and the concordance among the observers, Kappa = 0.70.

Style of childrearing perceived. A self-administered questionnaire is used, based on the Parental Bonding Instrument of Parker [28].

Development of the child. The cognitive and psychomotor development by means of the Bayley scales of Infant Development is tested [29]. The social development, through the appraisal scale of the Social Development is studied [10].

Perinatal Complications. These are detected by means of the scale of Perinatal Complications [30].

Diagnosis of Depressive Disorder

Existence and severity of postpartum depression. The disorder should be initiated during the first six postpartum months, evaluated from the clinical interviews and the PSE. These probable cases are considered by a board of four psychiatrists and, by consensus, the final diagnosis of depression is obtained according to the Finley-Jones criteria [31], as well as its severity, based on the scale of Social Adaptation. Four degrees are obtained: 1. isolated symptoms; 2. depressive syndrome with low interference; 3. depressive syndrome with moderate interference and 4. depressive syndrome with serious interference. The ones which score two or more will take part in the control group.

Duration of the postpartum depression. The duration of the depression, which is considered the most representative and reliable factor, is calculated in days (TDEP) at the sixth and twelfth month. This value is used in the statistical analysis.

Evaluations

The visits to the mother and child are carried out, in different sessions, by two interviewers, both blind to the results of the other explorations. On the third day, at the hospital, the questionnaire of sociodemographical data is completed, taking into account the clinical status of the mother and the style of childrearing perceived. Her clinical status is re-evaluated at the first, third, sixth, twelfth and twenty-eighth month. The interaction between the mother and the child will be evaluated at the first, sixth and twelfth month. The cognitive and psychomotor development of the child is evaluated at the sixth, twelfth and twenty-eighth month. The social development is assessed at the twelfth and twenty-eighth month. All these visits are at home of the mother, except the last wich is achieved at the hospital again.

RESULTS

Evolution of the Sample

The sample was selected out of 205 women; 35 (17%) did not conclude the first part of the study (six first months). The cases group was obtained from this sample (n = 23); the control group (n = 37) was selected at random. The final sample corresponds to those 60 women. Twelve months later 58 were interviewed, contact was lost with two of the control group. Finally, at the twenty-eighth month, the sample was comprised by 43 women (there were six losses in the control group, four in the cases group and, with the objective of establishing the existence of a differed effect of the depression on the development of the child, other five women were eliminated because they remained depressed after the year).

Sociodemographical Characteristics (Depressed vs Non-Depressed)

The average age of the women is 26 years (rank: 17-39 years). Most part of them are married (88.3%). The 41.6% has primary studies, the 33.3% secondary studies and the 25% university studies. The 60% does not have a remunerated job. The 65% of the women have intermediate economic incomes. There are not significant differences with regard to sociodemographical characteristics among the depressed mothers and those of the control group. In addition, no difference was found in the selected sample (n = 205) and the excluded one (n = 128). In conclusion, it is a sample of low social risk.

Severity and Duration of the Postpartum Depression

The 69.6% of the depressed mothers presented moderate and the 8.6% serious interference. The 65.2% of the depressed mothers kept being depressed six months later, the 43.4% twelve months later and finally, the 21.7% continued being depressed longer than a year, reaching the most part of them the twenty-eight months. The average duration of the postpartum depression, assessed on a year, was 26.3 weeks.

Statistical Analysis

Analysis Univariate

The possible relations, among the maternal variables (duration of the postpartum depression, style of childrearing) and those corresponding to the development of the child are individually studied. Moreover, the association between the duration of the postpartum depression and the style of childrearing is analysed.

Postpartum depression and development of the child. The cognitive development at six months is significantly lower in the children of depressed mothers (depressed: 101.8 vs non-depressed: 108.2; $p = 0.04$). The score in the social development of the children of depressed mothers is significantly lower at twelve months (depressed: 5.7 vs non-depressed: 7.1; $p = 0.01$).

Duration of the postpartum depression and development of the child (table I). The cognitive development of the children at the twenty-eight months is negatively influenced by the duration of the maternal depression during the first year. Besides, a negative association exists between the duration of the depression in the first six months and a lower social development of the child at the age of one year old.

Duration of the postpartum depression and style of childrearing (table II). A significant relation between the duration of the depression and a style of childrearing low in affection and care is observed at the twelfth month.

The style of childrearing perceived by the mothers is analysed and non-significant differences are obtained between those who get depressed and the ones who do not (affectionate style $p = 0.52$, overprotective style $p = 0.84$ and restrictive of liberty style $p = 0.17$).

Evolution in the style of childrearing between depressed and non-depressed mothers. A 43.47% and a 30.43% of the depressed mothers increase, respectively, the scores of style of childrearing low in affection and care, against an 8.10% of the non-depressed mothers.

Style of childrearing and development of the child (table III). A lower affection in the style of childrearing is associated to a lower cognitive and social development of the child during the first year, while the psychomotor development is only negatively influenced during the first six months. A lower cognitive and social development is evidenced at the age of one, when lack of care prevails in the style of childrearing. Lower social development is also evidenced at the twenty-eight month.

Variables of confusion and development of the child. None of the variables studied, neither maternal nor those related to the child, presents an effect on the development during the period of study.

Table I. Relation between the duration of the postpartum depression of the mother until the sixth month (TDEP 6 m) and the twelfth month (TDEP 12 m), and the scores of the development of the child (cognitive, psychomotor and social) provided by the correlation coefficients of Pearson (r).

	TDEP 6 m	TDEP 12 m	n
COGNI 6 m	-0.24	-----	60
COGNI 12 m	-0.13	-0.07	58
COGNI 28 m	-0.29*	-0.38**	43
MOTOR 6 m	0.04	-----	60
MOTOR 12 m	0.02	0.18	58
MOTOR 28 m	-0.26	-0.22	43
SOC 12 m	-0.34*	-0.30	36
SOC 28 m	0.04	0.01	48

* = $p < 0.05$; ** = $p < 0.01$

Table II. Relation between the duration of the postpartum depression of the mother until the sixth month (TDEP 6 m) and twelfth month (TDEP 12 m), and the style of childrearing provided by the correlation coefficients of Pearson (r).

	TDEP 6 m	TDEP 12 m	n
SRLA 6 m	0.20	-----	60
SRLC 6 m	0.23	-----	60
SRLA 12 m	0.38**	0.31*	58
SRLC 12	0.44**	0.45**	58

*= $p < 0.05$; ** = $p < 0.01$

Table III. Relation between the style of childrearing of the mother at the sixth and twelfth month, and the development (cognitive, psychomotor and social) of the child at the sixth, twelfth and twenty-eighth month provided by the correlation coefficients of Pearson (r).

	SRLA 6 m	SRLC 6 m	SRLA 12 m	SRLC 12 m	n
COGNI 6 m	-0.39**	-0.09	-----	-----	60
COGNI 12 m	-0.25	-0.25	-0.36**	-0.28*	58
COGNI 28 m	-0.14	-0.02	-0.21	-0.07	43
MOTOR 6 m	-0.27*	0.14	-----	-----	60
MOTOR 12 m	0.01	-0.19	-0.10	-0.15	58
MOTOR 28 m	-0.16	0.20	-0.17	0.09	43
SOC 12 m	-0.35**	-0.21	-0.50***	-0.46***	
36 SOC 28 m	-0.12	-0.33*	-0.12	-0.38**	43

* = p < 0.05; ** = p < 0.01; *** = p < 0.001

Analysis Multivariate

First, it is carried out an analysis of multiple linear regression with all the variables and their interactions (saturated model) and subsequently an analysis of linear regression at intervals, which is contributed by the model of predicting variables for every moment in which the development of the child is evaluated.

The clearest factor related to the cognitive development of the child during the first year of life is the style of childrearing, therefore, low affection during the first year of life seems to be determinant in a lower level of cognitive development in the children (at month sixth: n = 60, R^2 = 0.15, SRLA 6 m, t = 3.2, p = 0.002; at month twelfth: n = 58, R^2 = 0.13, SRLA 12 m, t = 2.8, p = 0.007).

The duration of the postpartum depression does not show any connection with the cognitive development of the child during the first twelve months. Nevertheless, it is observed that, with regard to the differed effect of the maternal depression, the interaction of the duration of the depression of the mother during the twelve first months and a style of childrearing low in affection in that period of time, is negatively associated with the cognitive development of the child at the age of twenty-eight months (n = 43, R^2 = 0.27, TDEP 12 m x SRLA 12 m, t = 3.9, p < 0.001).

Differences in the psychomotor development have not been found. The maternal factor that keeps a more constant relation with the level of psychomotor development of the child is the style of childrearing low in affection (at month sixth: n = 60, R^2 = 0.16, SRLA 6 m, t = 2.9, p = 0.005; at month twenty-eighth: n = 43, R^2 = 0.11, SRLA 12 m, t = 2.3, p = 0.02), although that relation seems to disappear at the year.

The social development of the child does not seem to have significant relation with the duration of the depression of the mother, but it does with the style of childrearing. Thus, at twelve months the social development of the child has a relation not only with the style of childrearing low in affection but also with the style of childrearing low in care (n = 36, R^2 = 0.34, SRLA 12 m, t = 2.5, p = 0.01, SRLC 12 m, t = 2.1, p = 0.04), then, the twenty-eight months will be associated only with the style of childrearing low in care during the first twelve months (n = 43, $R^2 = 0.10$, SRLC 12 m, t = 2.1, p = 0.03).

DISCUSSION

Methods

The problem of the sample is its small size. Most of the works present a similar sample [6,17-19,32-36]. A similar percentage of losses exists in all the studies of prospective and longitudinal design [10,17,21,37]. The percentage of mothers with postpartum depression (13.5%) is comparable to other studies [1,2,21,38].

The diagnostic criteria of depression used has a great reliability and validity of structure [31,39,40]. The PSE is used in many of the epidemiological studies to present a complete psychopathologic analysis and high reliability [41-43] and validity [39,40]. The duration of the postpartum depression is considered the most reliable and representative indicator for this kind of follow-up studies. The existence or not of depression or its severity, as it happens in other works [10,21,36], does not show, at any moment, the duration and the potential effect on the interaction with her child. The Bayley scales of Development are extensively translated and adapted in several countries, offering a high validity and reliability [29]. The scale for the Social Development of the child elaborated by Stein presents a great reliability, being used in studies of similar design [13].

In spite of the difficulty which involves the evaluation of the style of childrearing, the most adequate and sensitive method is the direct observation [6,7,32,34]. There are studies where the appraisal of the style of childrearing is performed by the mother by means of self-administered questionnaires [37,44]. The information of these questionnaires can be influenced by diverse maternal factors, such as the depression, losing objectivity.

Uniformity, respect to the moment in order to value the interaction mother-child, does not exist. Some works study a significant but non-defining moment of the day [20], others are centred on the structured [6,10] or non-structured game [6,7,45]. On the other hand, some studies assess the interaction of more specific moments in the care of the child, such as the diet [32,45]. The period in which the interaction of the mother-child is assessed is, sometimes, shorter than five minutes [7,46].

Style of Childrearing of the Mother

Relation between the type of childrearing perceived by the mother and the development of postpartum depression is not observed. Gotlib relates the postpartum depression with an over-protective and low in affection style of childrearing perceived by the mother. This is a retrospective study, the diagnosis is carried out through questionnaires and the state of the interviewed can alter the result [47]. In another study it is obtained a relation between depressive symptoms at the sixth postpartum month and a style of childrearing with great restriction of freedom, and not with a style of childrearing low in affection or high in overprotection [28].

The depressed mothers, and even more, those in whom the depression has a greater duration, develop a style of childrearing low in affection and care at the twelfth month. In this sense, Field indicates that the depressed mothers receive lower scores in all the interactions with the baby [46]. Some studies define the interaction of the depressed mother and her child, during the first months, as "negative" [7,48-50]. Numerous studies describe in the mothers with postpartum depression conducts less emotional towards their children [10,32,45,51,52]. Lyons-Ruth observes that the maternal aspects improved after the treatment for the depression related to the expression of affection towards their children [20].

Cognitive, Psychomotor and Social Development of the Child

It is observed a relation between the duration of the postpartum depression during the first year and the cognitive development of the child at the twenty-eighth months. In a meta-analysis carried out by Beck it is indicated the existence of a long-term effect of the postpartum depression on the cognitive development of the child [53]. In this sense, Cogill observes, at the age of four years old, a lower cognitive development in the children of mothers who had postpartum depression, but the study does not value the duration of the depression [18]. In other works, this relation is limited to the mothers with a lower level of education [54] or when the child is a male [55]. Some studies describe a lower cognitive development in the children of mothers with postpartum depression, valued during the first months [19,56]. Murray provides that the children of mothers with postpartum depression present, at the ninth, as well as at the eighteenth month, a lower level of cognitive development. The lower cognitive development is related to the severity of the maternal depression in the ninth month, but this association disappears in subsequent months [21]. This author finds relation between the postpartum depression of the mother and a lower cognitive development of the male children at the eighteenth month [57]. Nevertheless, this relation is not found when the child is valued at the age of 5 years old, even taking into account the sex and the social status [58]. Hay observes that the children of mothers who suffered postpartum depression present, at the age of 11 years old, lower scores in the intellectual index. This difference is more significant in the males [59]. Kurstjens and Wolke obtain also this more significant association when the duration of the depression is bigger, if the child is a male, and depending on different social factors of risk [60].

From these results, it could be obtained a relation between a lower cognitive or intellectual development in the child in more advanced ages and the prior existence of postpartum depression in the mother. However uniformity, does not exist in the results and then, more studies should be carried out.

In relation to the differed effect obtained in our study about the postpartum depression and the style of childrearing on the child, authors like Murray, observe that the mothers with postpartum depression are less sensitive and negative towards their children. This interaction predicts a lower cognitive development at the eighteen months [57]. Stanley obtains that, the response of the mother in the interaction with her child at the two months, predicts the development of child. This association is not found in the postpartum depression [51]. The relation between the sensibility of the mother towards the child in the first months and the adjustment and cognitive development of the child, has already been reflected in previous studies [61,62], but it is needed more specific studies.

Whiffen and Gotlib do not find differences on the psychomotor development between the children of mothers with or without postpartum depression [19], as it happens in our case. Nevertheless, these authors only study the children until two months of age, and they only analyse the presence or absence of postpartum depression, without defining the time of duration of it. It can be affirmed that the influence of the postpartum depression on the psychomotor development of the child is scarcely studied, although it does not seem to be very relevant.

With respect to the sociability of the child, diverse authors find that the children of mothers with postpartum depression present at the eighteen months a lower sociability and a more insecure attachment with their mothers [10,21,63,64]. In this sense, Lyons-Ruth obtains an association between the depression and an insecure attachment of the child at the age of one year old [20]. However, when Murray analyses the effect of the duration of the postpartum depression, does not find any relation [21], something which does happen in our study. This relation is also observed in more advanced ages of the child [65]. In this same line, Murray obtains that the relationship of the child with their mother at the age of five is mediated by the quality of the adjustment at the eighteen months [66]. Campbell and Cohn, on the contrary, do not find relation between the quality of the adjustment mother-child and the presence or duration of the postpartum depression [67]. Hopkins does not find either, a relation between the postpartum depression and a lower sociability of the child, although in this case, the study of the sociability is performed in a very premature moment, the second month of life [68].

The importance of the style of childrearing on the social development of the child, found in our study, is related to the significance of the stimulation, sensibility and maternal contact during the first year and a half of life on the social development of the child, something already indicated by other authors [69,70]. In this sense, Righetti describes the mothers with postpartum depression as less affectionate with their children and these more insecure with their mothers at the age of eighteen months [63].

CONCLUSION

1. The postpartum depression appears in a 13.5% of the sample studied. There are not found sociodemographical differences among depressed and not depressed women.
2. The duration of the depression is related to a style of childrearing low in affection and care, at least during the twelve months after the childbirth.
3. The duration of the depression of the mother does not exercise an effect on the development of the child in the first year. The style of childrearing low in affection is negatively associated with the cognitive, psychomotor and social development of the child in the first year, although in the case of the psychomotor development, the association is not maintained at the year.

4. The interaction of the duration of the depression of the mother and a style of childrearing low in affection during the first year is negatively associated with the cognitive development of the child at the twenty-eight months.

Positive Aspects of the Study

This longitudinal and prospective study permits a follow-up period and a frequency in the evaluations to detect changes in the mother and in the child. This diagnosis of depression is considered sensitive and reliable, being the duration of it, the most representative and reliable criteria for a follow-up study. The diverse variables are evaluated by different observers, avoiding slants in the observation. Finally our work studies the influence of the childrearing on the development of the child.

Limitations of the Study

The small size of the sample and the percentage of losses, similar in most of the studies, limit the results. The evaluation of the style of childrearing, although carried out by means of the observation method as more objective procedure, presents difficulties due to the complexity of this variable. The fact of being observed by an external evaluator could influence the normal behaviour of the mother. About the design of the work, this does not permit to provide a causality direction, being this limitation typical in the studies of observational nature.

Clinical Implications

The birth of a child involves important changes in the mother, as well as in the father, being able to reach the existence of a postpartum depression. This fact, produces in the mother a different attitude and conduct towards her child, this is reflected in a more negative style of childrearing, based on lower expressions of affection. All this can negatively influence the development of the child in so crucial and early ages, as it is the two first years and a half of life. The significance of this kind of results should be kept in mind at the moment of designing sociosanitary politics directed to the prevention and early intervention of this situation.

REFERENCES

[1] Cox, JL; Connor, Y; Kennedy, RE. Prospective study of the psychiatric disorders of childbirth. *British Journal of Psychiatry*, 1982 140, 111-117.
[2] Kumar, R; Robson, K.A. Prospective study of emotional disorders in childrearing women. *British Journal of Psychiatry*, 1984 144, 35-47.

[3] O´Hara, MW; Neunaber, DJ; Zekoski, EM. Prospective study of postpartum depression: prevalence, course and predictive factors. *Journal of Abnormal Psychology*, 1984 93, 158-175.

[4] Cooper, PJ; Campbell, FA; Day, A; Kennerly, H; Bond, A. Non-pschicotic psychiatry disorder after child birth: A prospective study of prevalance, incidence, course and nature. *British Journal of Psychiatry*, 1988 152, 799-806.

[5] Murray, L; Carothers, AD. The validation of the Edinburgh Postnatal Depression Scale on a comunity sample. *British Journal of Psychiatry*, 1990 157, 288-290.

[6] Cohn, JF; Matias, R; Tronick, EZ; Connell, D; Lyons-Ruth, D. Face-to-face interactions of depressed mothers and their infants. In: Tronick EZ, Field T editors. *Maternal Depression and Infant Disturbance*. San Francisco: Jossey Bass; 1986; 31-45.

[7] Field, T; Healy, B; Goldstein, S; Guthertz, M. Behavior-state matching and synchrony in mother-infant interactions in nondepressed versus depressed dyads. *Developmental Psychology*, 1990 26, 7-14.

[8] Uddenberg, N. Reproductive adaptation in mother and daughter. A study of personality development and adaptation to motherhood. *Acta Psychiatrica Scandinavica*, 1974 suppl 254, 1-115.

[9] Bromet, EJ; Cornely, PJ. Correlates of depression in mother of young children. *Journal of the American Academy Child Psychiatry*, 1984 23, 335-342.

[10] Stein, A; Gath, DH; Bucher, J; Bond, A; Day, A; Cooper, PJ. The relationship between post-natal depression and mother-child interaction. *British Journal of Psychiatry*, 1991 158, 46-52.

[11] Weissman, MM; Paykel, ES; Klerman, GL. The depressed woman as a mother. *Social Psychiatry*, 1972 7, 98-108.

[12] Clarke-Stewart, KA. Interactions between mothers and their young children: characteristics and consequences. *Monographs of the Society for Research in Child Development*, 1973 38, serial n° 153.

[13] Murray, L; Cooper, PJ. Effects of postnatal depression on infant development. *Archives of Disease in Childhood*, 1997 77, 99-101.

[14] Cooper, PJ; Tomlinson, M; Swartz, L; Woolgar, M; Murray, L; Molteno, CH. Post-partum depression and mother-infant relationship in a South African peri-urban. *British Journal of Psychiatry*, 1999 175, 554-558.

[15] Mills, M; Puckering, C; Pound, A; Cox, A. What is it about depressed mothers that influencies their children's functioning?. In: Stevenson JE, editor. *Recent research developmental psychopathology*. Oxford: Pergamon Press; 1985; 11-17.

[16] Williams, H; Carmichael, A. Depression in mothers in a multi-ethnic urban industrial municipality in Melbourne. Aetiological factors and effects on infants and preschool children. *Journal of Child Psychology and Psychiatry*, 1985 26, 277-288.

[17] Wrate, RM; Rooney, AC; Thomas, PF; Cox, JL. Postnatal depression and child development. A three-year follow-up study. *British Journal of Psychiatry*, 1985 14, 622-627.

[18] Cogill, SR; Caplan, HL; Alexandra, H; Robson, K; Kumar, R. Impact of postnatal depression on cognitive development in young children. *British Medical Journal*, 1986 292, 1165-1167.

[19] Whiffen, VE; Gotlib, IH. Infants of postpartum depressed mothers: temperament and cognitive status. *Journal of Abnormal Psychology*, 1989 98, 274-279.

[20] Lyons-Ruth, K; Connell, DB; Grunebaum, HU; Botein, S. Infants at social risk: maternal depression and family support services as mediators of infant development and security of attachment. *Child Development*, 1990 61, 85-98.

[21] Murray, L. The impact of postnatal depression on infant development. *Journal of Child Psychology and Psychiatry*, 1992 33, 543-361.

[22] Slade, P. Treating postnatal depression: A psychological approach for health care practitioners. *British Journal of Clinical Psychology*, 2000 39, 427-428.

[23] Lagerberg, D. Secondary prevention in child health: effects of psychological intervention, particulary home visitation, on children's development and other outcome variables. *Acta Paediatrica*, 2000 suppl 434, 43-52.

[24] Elliot, SA; Leverton, TJ; Sanjack, M; Turner, H; Cowmeadow, P; Hopkins, J; Bushnell, D. Promoting mental health after childbirth: A controlled trial of primary prevention of postnatal depression. *British Journal of Clinical Psychology*, 2000 39, 223-241.

[25] Wing, JK; Cooper, JE; Sartorius, N. *Measurement and Classification of Psychiatric Symptoms*. Cambridge: Cambridge University Press; 1974.

[26] Gómez Beneyto, M. *Scale of social adaptation* (unplished). Valencia; 1988.

[27] Parker, G; Tupling, H; Brown, LB. A parental bonding instrument. *British Journal of Medicine and Psychology*, 1979 52, 1-10.

[28] Gómez-Beneyto, M; Pedrós, A; Tomás, A; Aguilar, K; Leal, C. Psychometric properties of parental bonding instrument in a spanish sample. *Social Psychiatry and Psychiatric Epidemiology*, 1993 28, 252-255.

[29] Bayley, N. *Bayley scales of infant development*. New York: Psychological Corporation; 1969.

[30] Littman, B; Parmelee, AH. *Manual for the obstetric and postnatal complications scales*. Los Angeles: University of California; 1974.

[31] Finlay-Jones, R; Brown, GW; Duncan-Jones, P; Harris, T; Murphy, E; Prudo, R. Depression and anxiety in the community: replicationing the diagnosis of a case. *Psychological Medicine*, 1980 10, 445-454.

[32] Livingood, AB; Daen, P; Smith, BD. The depressed mother as a source of stimulation for her infant. *Journal of Clinical Psychology*, 1983 39, 369-375.

[33] Uddenberg, N; Englesson, I. Prognosis of postpartum mental disturbance. A propective study of primiparous women and their 4 1/2-year-old children. *Acta Psychiatrica Scandinavica*, 1978 58, 201-212.

[34] Field, TM; Sandberg, D; Garcia, R; Vega-Lahr, N; Goldstein, S; Guy, L. Pregnancy problems, postpartum depression and early mother-infant interactions. *Developmental Psychology*, 1985 21, 1152-1156.

[35] Ghodsian, M; Zajicek, E; Woldkind, S. A longitudinal study of maternal depression and child behavior problems. *Journal of Child Psychology and Psychiatry*, 1984 25, 91-109.

[36] Caplan, KL; Cogill, SR; Alexandra, H; Robson, K; Katz, R; Kumar, R. Maternal depression and the emotional development of the child. *British Journal of Psychiatry*, 1989 154, 818-822.

[37] Tamminen, T. The impact of mother's depression on her nursing experiences and attitudes during breastfeeding. *Acta Paediatrica Scandinavica*, 1988 suppl 77, 87-94.

[38] Cox, JL; Murray, D; Chapman, G. A controled study of the onset, duration and prevalence of postnatal depression. *British Journal of Psychiatry*, 1993 163, 27-31.

[39] Finlay-Jones, R; Brown, GW. Types of stressfull life event and the onset of anxiety and depressive disorders. *Psychological Medicine*, 1981 11, 803-815.

[40] Prudo, R ; Brown, GW ; Harris, T ; Dowland, J. Psychiatric disorder in a rural and an urban population: 2. Sensitivity to loss. *Psychological Medicine*, 1981 11, 601-616.

[41] Wing, JK; Birley, JL; Cooper, JE; Graham, P; Isaacs, AD. Reliability of a procedure for measuring and classifying "present psychiatric state". *British Journal of Psychiatry*, 1967 113, 499-515.

[42] Kendell, RE; Everitt, B; Cooper, JE; Sartorius, N; David, ME. Reliability of the Present State Examination. *Social Psychiatry*, 1968 3, 123-129.

[43] Luria, RE; Berry, R. Reliability and descriptive validity of PSE syndromes. *Archives of General Psychiatry*, 1979 36, 1187-1195.

[44] Raugh, VA; Wasserman, GA; Brunelli, SA. Determinants of maternal child-childrearing attitudes. *Journal of American Academy of Child and Adolescent Psychiatry*, 1990 29, 375-381.

[45] Fleming, AS; Ruble, DN; Flett, G; Shaul, DL. Postpartum adjustment in first-time mothers: relations between mood, maternal attitudes and mother-infant interactions. *Developmental Psychology*, 1988 24, 71-81.

[46] Field, TM; Healy, B; Goldstein, S; Perry, S; Bendell, D; Schanberg, S; Zimmerman, EA; Kuhn, C. Infants of depressed mothers show "depressed" behavior even with nondepressed adults. *Child Development*, 1988 59, 1569-1579.

[47] Gotlib, IH; Mount, JH; Cordy, NI; Whiffen, VE. Depression and perceptions of early parenting: a longitudinal investigation. *British Journal of Psychiatry*, 1988 152, 24-27.

[48] Cohn, JF; Tronick, EZ. Three-month-old infants' reaction to simulated maternal depression. *Child Development*, 1983 54, 185-193.

[49] Zekoski, EM; O'Hara, MW; Wills, KE. The effects of maternal mood on mother-infant interaction. *Journal of Abnormal Child Psychology*, 1987 15, 361-378.

[50] Bettes, BA. Maternal depression and motherese: temporal and intonational features. *Child Development*, 1988 59, 1089-1096.

[51] Stanley, C; Murray, L; Stein, A. The effect of postnatal depression on mother-infant interaction, infant response to the Still-face perturbation, and performance on an Instrumental Learning task. *Development and Psychopathology*, 2004 16, 1-18.

[52] Herrera, E; Reissland, N; Sheperd, J. Maternal touch and maternal-child directed speech; effects of depressed mood in the postnatal period. *Journal of Affective Disorders*, 2004 81, 29-39.

[53] Beck, CT. The effect of postpartum depression on child development: a meta-analysis. *Archives of Psychiatric Nursing*, 1998 12, 12-20.

[54] Hay, DF; Kumar, R. Interpreting the effects of mothers' postnatal depression on children's intelligence: a critique and reanalysis. *Child Psychiatry and Human Development*, 1995 25, 165-181.

[55] Sharp, D; Hay, D; Pawlby, S; Schmucher, G; Allen, H; Kumar, R. The impact of postnatal depression on boys intellectual development. *Journal of Child Psychology and Psychiatry*, 1995 36, 1315-1337.

[56] Lyons-Ruth, K; Zoll, D; Connell, D; Grunebaum, HU. The depressed mother and her one year old infant: enviroment, interaction, attachment and infant development. In: Tronick EZ, Field T editors. *Maternal depression and infant disturbance*. San Francisco: Jossey-Bass; 1986; 34.

[57] Murray, L; Fiori-Cowley, A; Hooper, R; Cooper, PJ. The impact of postnatal depression and associated adversity on early mother infant interactions and later infant outcome. *Child Development*, 1996 67, 2512-2526.

[58] Murray, L; Hipwell, A; Hooper, R; Stein, A; Cooper, PJ. The cognitive development of five-year-old children of postnatally depressed mothers. *Journal of Child Psychology and Psychiatry*, 1996 37, 927-936.

[59] Hay, DF; Pawlby, S; Sharp, D; Asten, P; Mills A; Kumar, R. Intellectual problems shown by 11-year-old children whose mothers had postnatal depression. *Journal of Child Psychology and Psychiatry*, 2001 42, 871-889.

[60] Kurtsjens, S; Wolke, D. Effects of maternal depression on cognitive development of children over the first 7 years of life. *Journal of Child Psychology and Psychiatry*, 2001 42, 623-636.

[61] Teti, DM; Gelfand, DM; Pompa, J. Depresed mothers' behavioral competence with their infants: Demographic and psychosocial correlates. *Development and Psychopathology*, 1990 2, 259-270.

[62] Isabella, RA; Belsky, J. Interactional synchrony and origins of infant-mother attachment: A replication study. *Child Development*, 1991 62, 373-384.

[63] Righetti-Veltema, M; Bousquet, A; Manzano, J. Impact of postpartum depressive symptoms on mother and her 18-month-old infant. *European Child and Adolescent Psychiatry*, 2003 12, 75-83.

[64] Edhborg, M; Lundh, W; Seimyr, L; Widstrom, AM. The parent-child relationship in the context of maternal depressive mood. *Archives of Women's Mental Health*, 2003 6, 211-216.

[65] Teti, DM; Gelfand, CM; Messinger, DS; Isabella, R. Maternal depression and quality of early attachment: an examination of infants, pre-schoolers, and their mothers. *Developmental Psychology*, 1995 31, 364-376.

[66] Murray, L; Sinclair, D; Cooper, P; Ducournau, P; Turner, P; Stein, A. The socioemotional development of 5-year-old children of postnatally depressed mothers. *Journal of Child Psychology and Psychiatry*, 1999 40, 1259-1271.

[67] Campbell, SB; Cohn, JF. The timing and chronicity of postpartum depression: implications in infant development. In: Murray L, Cooper PJ editors. *Postpartum Depression and Child Development*. New York: Guilford Press; 1996.

[68] Hopkins, J. Postpartum depression: the syndrome and its relationship to stress, infant characteristics and social support. *Doctoral tesis. University of Pittsburgh*; 1984.

[69] Belsky, J. The determinants of parenting. *Child Development* 1984 55, 83-96.

[70] Egeland, B; Farber, EA. Infant-mother attachment: factors related to its development and changes over time. *Child Development*, 1984 55, 753-771.

Chapter VIII

A RETROSPECTIVE ACCOUNT OF DIFFICULTY COPING AND STRESSORS IN THE FIRST YEAR POSTPARTUM BY FIRST-TIME MOTHERS AND FATHERS

Stephen Matthey[*]
Department of Psychology, University of Sydney; and Sydney South West Area Health Service, Sydney, Australia.

ABSTRACT

Much of the work that documents new parents coping experiences is based upon small sample sizes, thus making it difficult to know the rate at which such experiences occur. This study combined qualitative and quantitative information on this issue.

First time parents (221 mothers; 179 fathers) were surveyed one year after the birth about their experiences of coping. Results showed that 24% of women and 10% of men had experienced at least one episode of difficulty coping for more than 2 weeks. For approximately half of these women and men the onset of these longer duration episodes occurred after six weeks postpartum. All mothers and fathers reported that adjusting to the change in their life had impacted on them. In addition, other frequently reported stressors included: baby-care issues and fatigue (mothers and fathers); household chores; infant illness; financial concerns; lack of support; a lack of confidence; and tension with family members (mothers). For men frequent stressors included work-related stress and concern for his partner. There were few differences in reported stressors between women experiencing longer episodes and short episodes of difficulty coping. These data

---

[*] Correspondence concerning this article should be addressed to Dr. Stephen Matthey, Sydney South West Area Health Service, Research Director: Infant, Child & Adolescent Mental Health Service, Area Mental Health (ICAMHS) Mental Health Centre (Level 1), Locked Bag 7103, Liverpool BC NSW 1871. Australia. ph: (02)9616 4262; Fax: (02) 9601 2773; e-mail: stephen.matthey@swsahs.nsw.gov.au.

complement the qualitative studies on the experiences of new mothers and fathers, by quantifying the frequency of perceived stressors. This information can be used to normalise the experiences of new parents when providing them with appropriate services. In addition, the data suggest that just screening for psychosocial difficulties at one time point (e.g., 6 weeks postpartum) will miss a considerable proportion of women or men who may have difficulty coping at a later date. The lack of discernible differences in stressors between women self-reporting difficulty coping for long and short durations lends some support to the questionable usefulness of just focusing on women meeting diagnostic criteria for a mood disorder.

Keywords: postnatal depression; fathers; mothers; distress

INTRODUCTION

The term postnatal depression (PND), while not a diagnostic category in DSM-IV, is usually confined to women (or men) who meet DSM-IV criteria for major or minor depression, and have an infant of less than 12 months old. While DSM-IV does have a postpartum onset specifier (within 4 weeks of the birth), this short time span is rarely used by clinicians and researchers alike.

The rate of PND, using these criteria, has consistently been found to be between 8% and 15% for women (O'Hara & Swain, 1996), and between 1.0% and 5.3% for men (Matthey, Barnett, Ungerer & Waters, 2000; Matthey, Barnett, Howie, & Kavanagh, 2003). Expanding the criteria to include DSM-IV anxiety disorders increases the rate of caseness to around 20% for women and 10% for men (Matthey et al, 2003).

The terms postnatal depression or anxiety, being based upon a symptomatology model that originates from a medical model, are equated by some as indicating a mental illness. While this term does not necessarily mean that the aetiology is organic (cf. Barnett, Matthey & Boyce, 1999), this view is often put forward as an argument against the use of such terms or labels. Creedy and Schochet (1996) consider that diagnosing a woman with postnatal depression, and basing treatment upon such a 'disorder', results in treatment which "induce a false-coping strategy because the cause of the problem is not addressed" (p.14). The view that the label PND is unhelpful for women, in that it either fails to capture the experience of women, or implies an organic/hormonal aetiology with resulting medical-type interventions (e.g., medication), has also been expressed by others, including Barclay and Kent (1998), Barclay and Lloyd (1996), Jebali (1993), Lewis and Nicolson (1998), Mauthner (1998), and Nicolson (1990; 1999).

These investigators report on the experiences of women in the first year without using such diagnostic labels. They paint a common picture of women coming to terms with the changes or losses they experience, a sense of isolation, lack of support from their partners and physical adjustments (e.g., pain, sleep deprivation). This picture is usually collected through in-depth interviews with a small number of women. Thus Nicolson (1990, 1999) interviewed 24 women; Lewis and Nicolson (1998) report on a sample of 12 women, Mauthner (1993; 1998; 1999) reports on samples of 20 and 40 women, Ugarizza (2002) on 30 women and Beck (1992) investigated the experiences of seven women with high levels of postnatal distress. A slightly larger study was undertaken by Brown, Lumley, Small and Astbury (1994) who reported on the experiences of 45 depressed and 45 non-depressed women.

With regard to fathers, small-scale qualitative studies (e.g., n = 15) have shown that men experience strain in their relationship with their partner and find fatherhood more difficult than they expected. Stressors include the sense of responsibility, settling a crying baby, the balancing of work and family demands and struggling for recognition as a father (Jordan, 1990; Barclay & Lupton, 1999; Lupton & Barclay, 1997).

While such qualitative studies on mothers and fathers provide us with a much better understanding of the difficulties they experience than the quantitative studies focusing on rates of diagnostic disorders, they do not describe how many women and men experience different stressors. We do not know, for example, what percentage of new mothers or fathers experience a sense of isolation or family tension in the first year postpartum that they consider contributed to any difficulty they had in coping. In part this is because the studies use small sample sizes, a necessity of qualitative research; in part it may also reflect a philosophy behind qualitative research, that research findings should not be "arrived at by means of statistical procedures or other means of quantification" (Strauss & Corbin, 1990; p.17). There is, however, an argument for reporting both individual's experiences, as well as the rate at which these events are experienced. By knowing which stressors are commonly reported by new parents, and which are less frequent, we can feed this back to new, or expectant, parents, thereby normalising some experiences. It can also serve to help health professionals plan preventive work. Clearly there will be more demand to address common stressors in postpartum services than infrequent ones; at the same time there needs to be an awareness of the infrequent stressors to ensure that women, and men, do not fall through the net.

Aims of the Study

This study utilised a survey sent to women and men at 1 year postpartum. The survey aimed to collect data about their beliefs as to the aetiology of any episodes of self-defined distress they had experienced in that first year, as well as their recollection as to the onset and duration of these episodes. As such it is important to emphasise that the parents' perceptions, and reports, of their distress are not considered equivalent to any diagnostic category, such as major or minor depression.

METHOD

Participants

English-speaking couples expecting their first child who attended antenatal classes at a public hospital in South West Sydney, Australia, were recruited for the study, the main aim of which was to investigate the effectiveness of a postnatal distress prevention programme (see Matthey, Kavanagh, Howie, Barnett & Charles, 2004). This study followed the couples through the transition to parenthood, with assessments antenatally (at recruitment) and again at 6 weeks and 6 months postpartum, with the Experiences Survey being completed at one year postpartum. Mean age for the women was 27.1 years (S.D. = 4.2) and for the men 29.0 years (S.D. = 4.6). Of the women 48.7% had 11 years of education, and of the men 59.1% had this level of education. A further 21.7% of women and 14.3% of men had a tertiary education qualification (i.e. at least 16 years of education).

Measure

The 'Experiences Survey' was devised by the author. It consisted of five questions: Q1: an open-ended question about what had made becoming a parent enjoyable or easy; Q2: an open-ended question about what had made becoming a parent difficult or unenjoyable; Q3: whether she/he had found it difficult to cope since the baby was born, with five options ('No'; 'Yes – for less than a week'; 'Yes, for between 1 and 2 weeks'; 'Yes, for a period longer than 2 weeks' (duration then specified); and 'Yes, for several periods' (each duration specified, up to a maximum of three such periods); Q4: If she/he answered 'yes' to Q3, to specify how old the baby was when she/he started having difficulty coping (if more than one episode, to document this for each episode); Q5: a checklist of 21 possible stressors that may have contributed to the woman/man feeling stressed. These were based upon the literature, and are subsumed under the categories shown in Table 2.

All responses to the open-ended stressors question (Q2) were coded. Two investigators then reviewed these responses, and collapsed them into a smaller number of categories. For example, responses stating that the infant was unsettled, or that there had been feeding difficulties, were grouped into a 'baby-care' stressor.

Discriminant validity for this measure was determined by analysing diagnostic interview data at six week postpartum.

Procedure

The Experiences Survey was mailed at 1 year postpartum to all participants who had responded to the previous assessment at six months postpartum. The surveys were sent separately to the women and men, and each contained a stamped-addressed envelope for return to the research team.

RESULTS

Participants

From the original sample of 441 couples recruited in pregnancy, 221 women (50%) and 179 men (40.5%) responded to this survey at 12 months postpartum. These represented 71.3% of women and 57.7% of the men who had participated at the six-month assessment point. Some respondents failed to complete all 5 questions on the Experiences Survey. Thirteen women and seven men completed one or other of the open-ended stressor question or checklist question, but not both. Given that the results combine their responses to these two questions, they have been expressed as a percentage of the total surveys received.

Difficulty Coping

Table 1 details the percentage of women and men reporting difficulty coping in the first year postpartum. Half of the 23.6% of women, and also of the 9.8% of men, who reported an episode of more than 2 weeks duration stated that this episode started after six weeks postpartum.

Table 1. Percentages of Self-Reported Periods of Difficulty Coping in the First Year Postpartum:

Difficulty coping category	Mothers (N = 221)	Fathers (N = 179)
No difficulty coping	26.7	52.5
1 period for less than 1 week	27.1	22.3
1 period, between 1 & 2 weeks	11.8	10.6
Several periods, none more than 2 weeks long	10.0	0
At least 1 period for more than 2 weeks*	23.6[a]	9.8[b]

Note: Each column does not tally to 100% due to missing data on a few women and men.
* Includes those who report several episodes, of which at least one was more than 2 weeks long.
[a]Range 3-52 weeks duration (52 = still ongoing); [b]Range 4-56 weeks duration (56=still ongoing).

Responses to the Open-Ended Questions and Checklist

There were initially over 110 stressors reported by the men and women to the open-ended question. Re-classification of these into categories resulted in 24 stressors being coded. Rates of responses to each category were combined for the open-ended question and the checklist, as shown in Table 2. On one stressor only, that of baby care issues (which includes unsettled behaviour and feeding difficulties), was there a statistically significant difference in the rate between women reporting being distressed for more than 2 weeks and those distressed for 2 weeks or less (91.5% vs 46.8%; χ^2 (1,141) = 24.61, $p < .001$, $\phi = 0.42$). Lacking support approached significance in this comparison (12.8% vs 4.3%; χ^2 (1,141) = 2.27, $p = .06$, $\phi = 0.13$). For men also only one stressor was reported significantly more often by those feeling distressed for more than 2 weeks compared to those feeling distressed for 2 weeks or less - that of work-related stress (29.4% vs 8.8%; χ^2 (Fisher's exact) (1, 74) = 4.77, $p < .05$, $\phi = 0.21$). Cramer's phi values indicate that these associations range from low (0.1-0.29) to moderate (0.3- 0.49) (Matthey, 1998).

Table 2 also shows the significant differences in reported stressors between mothers and fathers.

Table 2. Rates of Reported Stressors, Combining Responses to the Open-Ended Question and the Checklist: Mothers and Fathers.

Stressor	Total sample		φ
	Mothers (N = 221)	Fathers (N = 179)	
Adjusting to the new situation (including the sense of responsibility)	100	100	
The baby had sleep, settling or feeding difficulties	66.2	50.3**	0.16
I was exhausted	54.1	36.3***	0.17
I was trying to do too many household chores	29.7	6.1***	0.30
Feeling isolated or lonely	25.7	3.9***	0.30
My baby was ill	20.3	17.3	
I lacked confidence in caring for the baby[1]	19.8	9.5**	0.14
Worried about money	19.4	22.9	
A lack of support	19.4	6.7***	0.18
There was tension with family members	16.2	6.1**	0.16
My health was poor	14.4	6.7*	0.12
Our marriage was suffering difficulties	13.5	6.1*	0.12
I was stressed at work[2]	11.7	24.6**	0.17
Someone I loved was very ill or died	5.4	4.5	
My partner was having difficulty coping	5.4	21.2***	0.24
Feeling bored	5.0	1.7	
There were problems with the delivery	4.1	6.1	
I am prone to feeling depressed anyway	2.3	1.7	
My partner's physical health was poor	0.5	8.4***	0.20
Worried may be pregnant again	0.5	-	
Partner's shopping habits	-	0.5	
Finding adequate daycare	1.0	-	
Renovating/moving house	1.0	-	
Baby growing up too quickly	1.0	-	
Being a single parent	0.5	-	
Baby responding to others more than to self	0.5	-	
Caring for more than 1 child[3]	0.5	-	

*$p < .05$; **$p < .01$; ***$p < .001$; women vs men (phi values of 0.3 or higher indicate a moderate degree of association - Matthey, 1998)

[1] This item only included for a subsample of those surveyed (total N = 91 women and 83 men)

[2] The percentage of women that this item applied to (i.e., were working) is not known.

[3] While all participants were first-time parents, one mother cared for another child on a regular basis.

LIMITATIONS

The checklist component of the Experiences Survey is not a definitive list of all possible stressors that could be experienced by new parents, which in part is why this was preceded by the open-ended stressor question. However, it is accepted that neither method can be sure of capturing all possible stressors that women might acknowledge on a self-report survey. It is likely that face-face in-depth interviews provide a richer understanding of not only the types of stressors, but also how these stressors affect women and men differently. However, as previously mentioned, by necessity such interviews cannot be undertaken on large samples of women and men. We feel the survey used therefore complements both the qualitative and quantitative research findings of other investigators.

That no formal psychometric properties of questions 3 and 4 in the survey have been investigated (eg., test-retest reliability; concurrent validity) is acknowledged as a limitation.

The rates of difficulty coping for more than two weeks or more (21.7% for women; 9.7% for men) should not be compared to diagnostic rates of postnatal depression in other studies, for several reasons. Firstly, this study did not use a diagnostic interview, but a self-report measure of difficulty coping. Secondly, the time frame is different - diagnostically the time frame is 2 weeks or more; in this study we used more than two weeks. Thirdly, only around half the original sample of women and men recruited antenatally responded to this survey at 12 months postpartum – there may therefore be a bias with respect to likelihood of staying in the study and experiences of coping. Fourthly, diagnostic rates tend to only assess depression. This study used whatever the adult considered defined 'difficulty coping' - thus it could include concepts such as anxiety and distress. The rationale for this is very much along the lines of those arguing that we need to understand women's experiences from their perspective (e.g., Mauthner, 1998). Whether or not a woman meets objective diagnostic criteria is not as relevant as whether a woman herself says she is having difficulty coping - it is this latter concept that should determine the offer of help from professionals, and not whether she meets criteria for a mental disorder. The same view also applies to the mental health of men.

DISCUSSION

The most frequently cited stressors associated with both women's and men's difficulties in coping in the first year postpartum were adjustment to their new situation, sleep, settling or feeding difficulties with their infant, and exhaustion. In addition, a substantial percentage of women (i.e., at least 20%) reported the following stressors: doing too many chores; feeling isolated or lonely; and her infant being sick. For men these other stressors were financial worries, stress at work, and concern for how his partner was coping. In addition, other frequent stressors for women (i.e., 10-19%) included a lack of confidence in caring for the baby, financial concerns, a lack of support, and tension with family members. For men the only additional frequent stressor was the health of his baby.

It is interesting that only one stressor was more prevalent for women (baby care issues) and men (work-related) reporting difficulty coping for two weeks or more compared to those with shorter periods of difficulty coping. This lends credence to investigators who believe focusing on women meeting diagnostic criteria for depression may be pathologising their condition. By simply focusing on such women it could be easy to (incorrectly) presume that women not meeting diagnostic criteria do not experience such stressors. As this study shows, this may be a false presumption. Clearly the experience of an event as stressful is an interaction of the event, the person's personality (e.g., coping style), and the context (e.g., the degree of support he/she receives). Given this, it is not surprising that for nearly all the stressors there is no simple relationship with reported duration of difficulty coping.

A similar percentage (40% approximately) of women and men report that the time of onset of an episode of distress that lasted more than two weeks was after six weeks postpartum. This is similar with the study of Brown et al (1994), who found that 55% of their women reported an onset of depression after three months postpartum. The importance of this finding is that much research conducted into rates of postnatal depression is done at 6 weeks postpartum. While self-reported distress is not pnd, this finding would suggest that clinicians and researchers need to keep in mind that it is likely that the onset of significant periods of distress can occur at any time in the first year postpartum. Thus assessing for such conditions at just one time point will likely fail to convey a full picture of women's experiences. In addition, it points to a need to continue to monitor a woman's mood during the first year postpartum as she has regular contact with the health services. As new events occur (e.g., teething; introduction of solids), and as environmental contexts may change (e.g., level of support may alter over time), so a mother, and possibly father, may experience a significant episode of difficulty coping. If we become too fixated on screening for distress in mothers only at one time point (e.g., the 6-week postnatal check-up) we are likely to miss the opportunity to offer professional support that may be helpful to the family at other times.

In the same way that a recent paper described the rate of expectant mothers' and fathers' postpartum concerns during pregnancy (Matthey, Morgan, Healey, Barnett, Kavanagh & Howie, 2002), so this study has documented the rate of reported stressors in a reasonable size sample of first time mothers and fathers in the first year postpartum. It is hoped that this information will prove helpful for clinicians conducting postpartum groups or services focusing on the experiences of new parents.

CONCLUSION

This study provides information as to the frequency of stressors in the first year postpartum for both mothers and fathers. Such information should prove useful for preventative services, as well as for parents who may feel reassured that their experiences are also experienced by substantial numbers of other parents. That baby-care stress is associated with longer periods of difficulty coping for women lends support to interventions aimed at reducing infant sleep and settle problems in order to also ameliorate postnatal distress in women (e.g., Hiscock & Wake, 2002). Whether there is a way of impacting on work-related stress for fathers to reduce the longer duration of difficulty coping for them remains to be seen.

ACKNOWLEDGMENTS

Prof. Bryanne Barnett
This project was funded by a grant from the Commonwealth Department of Health and Family Services (Research section), Australia, and Karitane, Australia.

REFERENCES

Barclay, L. & Kent, D. (1998). Recent immigration and the misery of motherhood: a discussion of pertinent issues. *Midwifery, 14*, 4-9.

Barclay, L. M. & Lloyd, B. (1996). The misery of motherhood: alternative approaches to maternal distress. *Midwifery, 12*, 136-139.

Barclay, L. & Lupton, D. (1999). The experiences of new fatherhood: a socio-cultural analysis. *Journal of Advanced Nursing, 29*, 1013-1020.

Barnett, B. E. W., Matthey, S., & Boyce, P. Migration and motherhood: a response to Barclay & Kent (1999). *Midwifery, 15*, 203-207.

Beck, C. T. (1992). The lived experience of postpartum depression: a phenomenological study. *Nursing Research, 41*, 166-170.

Brown, S., Lumley, J., Small, R. & Astbury, J. (1994). *Missing voices - the experience of motherhood*. Melbourne: Oxford University Press.

Creedy, D. & Shochet, I. (1996). Caring for women suffering depression in the postnatal period. *Australian and New Zealand Journal of Mental Health Nursing, 5*, 13-19.

Hiscock, H., & Wake, M. (2002). Randomised controlled trial of behavioural infant sleep intervention to improve infant sleep and maternal mood. *British Medical Journal, 324*, 1062-1065.

Jebali, C. (1993). A feminist perspective on postnatal depression. *Health Visitor, 66*, 59-60.

Jordan, P. L. (1990). Laboring for relevance: expectant and new fatherhood. *Nursing Research*, 39, 11-16.

Lewis, S. E. & Nicolson, P. (1998). Talking about early motherhood: recognizing loss and reconstructing depression. *Journal of Reproductive and Infant Psychology, 16*, 177-197.

Lupton, D. & Barclay, L. (1997). *Constructing fatherhood: discourses and experiences*. London: Sage Publications.

Matthey, S. (1998). p < .05. But is it *clinically* significant? Practical examples for clinicians. *Behaviour Change, 15*, 140-146.

Matthey, S., Barnett, B., Ungerer, J., Waters, B. (2000). Paternal and maternal depressed mood during the transition to parenthood. *Journal of Affective Disorders, 60*, 75-85

Matthey, S., Morgan, M., Healey, L., Barnett, B., Kavanagh, D.J. & Howie, P. Postpartum issues for expectant mothers and fathers. (2002). *Journal of Obstetrics, Gynecology and Neonatal Nursing, 31*, 428-435.

Matthey, S., Barnett, B.E.W., Howie, P & Kavanagh, D.J. (2003). Diagnosing postpartum depression in mothers and fathers: whatever happened to anxiety? *Journal of Affective Disorders, 74*, 139-147.

Matthey, S., Kavanagh, D. J., Howie, P., Barnett, B., Charles, M. (2004). Prevention of Postnatal Distress or Depression: An evaluation of an intervention at Preparation for Parenthood classes. *Journal of Affective Disorders, 79,* 113-126.

Mauthner, N. (1993). 1. Towards a feminist understanding of 'postnatal depression'. *Feminism and Psychology, 3,* 350-355.

Mauthner, N. S. (1998). "It's a woman's cry for help": a relational perspective on postnatal depression. *Feminism & Psychology, 8,* 325-355.

Mauthner, N. S. (1999). "Feeling low and feeling really bad about feeling low": Women's experiences of motherhood and postpartum depression. *Canadian Psychology, 40,* 143-161.

Nicolson, P. (1990). Understanding postnatal depression: a mother-centred approach. *Journal of Advanced Nursing, 15,* 689-695.

Nicolson, P. (1999). Loss, happiness and postpartum depression: The ultimate paradox. *Canadian Psychology, 40,* 162-178.

O'Hara, M.W. & Swain, A.M. (1996) Rates and risk of postpartum depression - a meta-analysis. *International Review of Psychiatry, 8,* 37-54.

Strauss, A. & Corbin, J. (1990). *Basics of qualitative research: Grounded theory procedures and techniques.* Newbury park, CA: Sage Publications.

Ugarriza, D. N. (2002). Postpartum depressed women's explanation of depression. *Journal of Nursing Scholarship, 34,* 227-233.

Chapter IX

ANIMAL MODELS OF POSTPARTUM DEPRESSION: STEROID HORMONE CONTRIBUTIONS AND ADULT NEUROGENESIS

*Jodi L. Pawluski, Amanda D. Green,
Cindy Barha and Liisa AM Galea**

Program in Neuroscience, Department of Psychology and Brain Research Center,
University of British Columbia, 2136 West Mall, Vancouver, BC, V6T 1Z4.

ABSTRACT

Postpartum depression (PPD) is a serious medical condition that affects more than 11 % of new mothers. The effects of PPD are debilitating to both the mother and her children. For example, longitudinal studies have revealed that women with untreated PPD have impaired cognitive ability, experience increased marital difficulties, and are more likely to abuse their children, and commit infanticide. In addition, children of mothers with PPD have an increased risk to develop depression or anxiety disorders in adulthood (Nomura et al., 2002), present with impaired cognitive, motor and social development (Murray and Cooper 1997; Nomura et al., 2002) and are less attached to their mothers during infancy (Righetti et al., 2005). The cause of postpartum depression is not known, but PPD and other pregnancy/postpartum-associated neuropsychiatric diseases such as post-partum psychosis have been suggested to be due to the profound hormone fluctuations during pregnancy and the postpartum period (Hendrick et al., 1998). Indeed, estradiol and cortisol/corticosterone are particularly involved in depression and given that there are large fluctuations in these steroid hormones across pregnancy and the post-partum period it may not be surprising that these hormone disturbances are related to the expression of post-partum depression. Furthermore,

---

* Correspondence concerning this article should be addressed to Liisa A.M. Galea, Ph.D., Associate Professor, The University of British Columbia, 2136 West Mall, Vancouver, B.C. V6T 1Z4 Phone: (604) 822-6536, Fax: (604) 822-6923, Email: lgalea@psych.ubc.ca.

estradiol and corticosterone have been shown to affect adult neurogenesis in the hippocampus. Adult hippocampal neurogensis is thought to play an important role in depression as chronic antidepressants upregulate hippocampal neurogenesis (Malberg et al., 2000), and animal models of depression show suppressed levels of neurogenesis (Jaako-Movits and Zharkovsky, 2005; Jayatissa, et al., 2006). The present review will focus on the role of the steroid hormones, estradiol and corticosterone, in the development and treatment of PPD, focusing on animal models of PPD which we have previously described and are presently developing. These animal models are based on estrogen-withdrawal across parturition (Galea et al., 2001) and elevated corticosterone levels during the postpartum (Brummelte et al, 2006). Understanding the etiology and treatment of this debilitating disorder is essential for determining how we can promote well-being in mothers and their children.

Keywords: Hormones, estradiol, cortisol, corticosterone, hippocampus, hippocampal neurogenesis, stress, depression, postparturition, pregnancy, HPA, HPG

INTRODUCTION

Postpartum depression (PPD) is a debilitating disease that affects approximately 11-13% of mothers (Altshuler et al., 2000; Georgiopoulos et al., 1999; O'Hara and Swain, 1996). This disease has well documented health consequences for the mother, child, and family; children of mothers with PPD have an increased risk to develop psychiatric disorders (Nomura et al., 2002), present with impaired cognitive, motor and social development (Murray and Cooper, 1997; Nomura et al., 2002) and are less attached to their mothers during infancy (Righetti et al., 2005). In addition, women who have depression during the postpartum are more likely to experience future episodes of depression (Cooper and Murray, 1995).

Intriguingly, women are twice as likely than men to suffer from major depression (Lehtinen and Joukamaa, 1994; Pearlstein et al., 1997), but only recently has research began to focus on the role of depression on the female brain and behaviour. Given that there is a sex difference in the incidence of depression, it may not be surprising that sex steroid hormones have been implicated as a mediator of depressive symptoms in women. In particular, hormones such as estradiol and progesterone, which are involved in the Hypothalamic-Pituitary-Gonadal axis (HPG) axis, and the hormone cortisol, which is involved in the Hypothalamic-Pituitary-Adrenal (HPA) axis, are associated with depression (Steiner et al., 2003; Swaab et al., 2005). The HPA axis is involved in responses to stress such that high levels of stress often result in elevated glucocorticoid levels and stress has been cited as a precipitating event prior to depression onset (Wolkowitz et al., 2001). Interestingly, the incidence of depression has been associated with fluctuations in estrogen levels (Douma et al., 2005; Steiner et al., 2003) and in stress/HPA axis reactivity (De Kloet, 2004). This is, perhaps, not suprising as there is known interactions between the HPG and HPA axes (Viau, 2002).

Animal models of depression in the adult female have found that the steroid hormones estradiol and corticosterone play a significant role in depressive symptomology (Dalla et al., 2004; Kalynchuk et al., 2004; Shively et al., 1997; Okada et al., 1997). Dalla et al (2004)

report that estradiol-deficit female mice (aromatase knockout (ArKO)), exhibit significant depressive-like symptoms compared to wild-type female mice. Shively et al (1997) report that chronic stress may result in depression by causing HPA axis and ovarian dysfunction in female primates. In addition, Kalynchuk et al (2004) have found that chronic high levels of corticosterone administered to adult male and female rats leads to an increase in depressive-like behaviour and is a potential model for the study of major depression in rodents (Gregus et al., 2005; Kalynchuk et al., 2004).

More recently, neural plasticity in the hippocampus has been associated with depression. Depressed patients can present with decreased hippocampal volume and impaired cognition; which is related to duration of illness and not age of subject (Sheline et al., 1999). While the cause of the reduced hippocampal volume is not known, there are suggestions that adult hippocampal neurogenesis may be reduced in depressed patients (Sheline, 2000). In particular, adult neurogenesis, which occurs in the dentate gyrus of the hippocampus, is increased by *chronic,* but not acute, treatment with antidepressants (Malberg et al., 2000), and elimination of adult hippocampal neurogenesis prevents the behavioral benefit of antidepressants in mice (Santarelli et al., 2003). This has led to the theory that an enhancement of hippocampal neurogenesis can alleviate depression and therefore the suppression of neurogenesis may lead to depression. In fact, in two different animal models of depression (olfactory bulbectomy and chronic mild stress) evidence suggests that adult hippocampal neurogenesis is significantly reduced (Jaako-Movits and Zharkovsky, 2005; Jayatissa, et al., 2006). Other factors that have been associated with depression, such as *chronic* stress and/or high-level corticosterone, also suppress neurogenesis (Huang and Herbert, 2005; Pham et al., 2003). Therefore, changes in hippocampal neurogenesis during adulthood may be an important marker in understanding the role of depression on the brain and subsequent behaviour.

Much less research has focused on the role of postpartum depression (PPD) on the mother and her offspring. The neural, hormonal and behavioral mechanisms behind these changes have yet to be fully understood. PPD and disorders associated with pregnancy and the postpartum have been suggested to be due to fluctuations in gonadal hormones (Hendrick et al., 1998) and/or changes in response to stress (and therefore the function of the HPA axis) associated with motherhood (O'Hara and Swain, 1996; Beck, 2001; Bernazzani et al., 1997; O'Hara et al., 1991). With regard to gonadal hormones, research has highlighted two significant alterations in the hormone profile during the postpartum that could precipitate depressive symptoms among susceptible women. The first alteration is the sharp drop in levels of the gonadal steroid hormones estradiol and progesterone. Estradiol and progesterone levels rise steadily during pregnancy due to placental production of these steroids (reviewed in Hendrick et al., 1998). In fact, estradiol increases 100-fold and progesterone increases 10-fold compared to maximal menstrual cycle levels (reviewed in Hendrick et al., 1998; Bloch et al., 2003). Removal of the placenta at delivery causes a precipitous drop in both estradiol and progesterone levels during the postpartum period (reviewed in Hendrick et al., 1998). This leads to the second alteration in the hormone profile during postpartum which is the prolonged hypogonadal state that occurs after parturition and lasts until restoration of ovulation and the menstrual cycle. Estradiol reaches early follicular levels by days 1 to 3 and progesterone by days 3 to 7 postpartum (Bloch et al., 2003) and they remain at low follicular levels for at least 40 days after parturition in nonlactating women and 160 days after parturition in lactating women (Perez, 1972). Therefore, the abrupt withdrawal and sustained low levels of gonadal steroid hormones during the postpartum may contribute to postpartum depression and postpartum mood disorders.

Pregnancy and the postpartum appear to be a time when there are significant changes in the function of the HPA axis and changes in the degree of perceived stress, which may relate to changes in postpartum mood. During pregnancy, cortisol has been shown to rise to at least three times the levels in nonpregnant women (Harris et al., 1994) and at parturition, the maternal HPA axis has been suggested to readjust as there is a loss of corticotropin releasing hormone (CRH) with the expulsion of the placenta (Carter et al., 2001). Furthermore, postpartum women reporting postpartum blues and postpartum depression have a delay in the recovery of normal HPA axis responding, as measured by changes in ACTH levels, compared to women with a normal psychological profile, regardless of whether they breast feed or not (Magiakou et al., 1996). Interestingly, others have found women who breast feed exhibit lower cortisol and behavioural responses to several types of stressors compared to women who bottle-feed their infants (Walker et al., 2004). An increase in the level of perceived stress with pregnancy and motherhood has also consistently been shown to contribute to postpartum depression (Beck, 2001; O'Hara and Swain, 1996; Bernazzani et al., 1997; O'Hara et al., 1991). For example, Beck (2001) reported childcare stress and life stress as two of the top five predictors of postpartum depression based on an meta-analysis of 84 studies published in the 1990s. In another interesting study Bloch et al. (2005) found that women with a history of PPD, exhibited higher levels of cortisol during a hormone regime mimicing pregnancy, indicating that women with a predisposition to PPD may have a more sensitive cortisol response to elevated estradiol and progesterone. More research is needed in understanding the changes in the HPA axis with pregnancy and the postpartum but it appears that stress, which is usually accompanied by elevated glucocorticoid levels, and irregular HPA axis functioning during the postpartum are contributors to postpartum blues and postpartum depression.

In order to understand the effects of hormone changes on the etiology and treatment of postpartum depression, we have developed two animal models of PPD based on either estradiol withdrawal in the mother after parturition, or increased corticosterone levels in the mother during the postpartum with the focus on the degree of 'depressive' behavior and alterations in hippocampal adult neurogenesis. The following review will focus on the animal models of postpartum depression developed in our laboratory: 'estradiol-withdrawal' model of PPD and the 'corticosterone-induced' model of PPD.

i. The Role of Estradiol in an Animal Model of PPD

The ovarian steroid hormones are well known modulators of mood and cognition, affecting numerous aspects of central nervous system functioning (McEwen, 2002). Estrogen in particular has widespread effects on the brain (Boulware and Mermelstein, 2005), and is a known "mood modifier" (Douma et al., 2005). Its dramatic fluctuations during pregnancy and the postpartum period may play a key role in developing postpartum depression (PPD)

(Spinelli, 2005). During the third trimester of pregnancy, endogenous estrogens (synthesized primarily from the placenta) increase 100 times normal levels, then return to pre-follicular levels within 5 days of parturition, and progesterone increases 10 fold (reviewed in Hendrick et al., 1998). This sustained rise and subsequent rapid decline in estrogen may precipitate depressive symptoms in vulnerable women (Hendrick et al., 1998; Studd and Panay, 2004; Douma et al., 2005) and has lead to the "estrogen withdrawal" hypothesis of PPD. This hypothesis has garnered growing support from both clinical studies (Sichel et al., 1995; Gregoire et al., 1996; Ahokas et al., 2001) and more recently animal models of PPD (Galea et al, 2001).

Clinical research suggests an important role for estrogen in depression (Studd and Panay, 2004). As mentioned previously, women have a much greater chance of developing major depressive disorders than men (Pearlstein et al., 1997), and studies suggest women report greater depression during times of a decline in gonadal hormone levels; including menopause, the premenstrual period, and the post-partum (Parry et al., 2003; Steiner et al., 2003; Studd and Panay, 2004). Estrogen's role in mediating post-partum depression is supported by its therapeutic efficacy; work has demonstrated that estrogen replacement can significantly alleviate PPD symptoms in subset of depressed women (Sichel et al., 1995; Gregoire et al., 1996; Ahokas et al., 2001). This work provides a clinical basis for the proposed connection between the postpartum withdrawal of estrogen and PPD.

Estrogen and progesterone together have also been proposed as mediators of postpartum depression. In an interesting study Bloch et al (2000) investigated mood after an experimental model of the hormone withdrawal period after parturition in women. In this model they administered estradiol and progesterone to women for 8 weeks to mimic the three main hormonal phases of pregnancy: elevated estradiol and progesterone levels during pregnancy, the sharp decline in hormonal levels at parturition, and the postpartum hypogonadal state (Bloch et al., 2000). They demonstrated that women with a history of PPD expressed more depressive symptoms compared to controls following the abrupt cessation of hormones (Bloch et al., 2000). This indicates that women with a history of PPD are more sensitive to estrogen and progesterone withdrawal. Together, these studies provide a basis for the proposed connection between the postpartum withdrawal of gonadal hormones, previous disposition to depression and PPD. Other researchers have also found an association between estradiol and progesterone levels and the development of PPD (Nott et al., 1976; Feksi et al., 1984; Abou-Saleh et al., 1998); whereas many others have not (Kuevi et al., 1983; O'Hara et al., 1991; Heidrich et al., 1994; Harris et al., 1996; Buckwalter et al., 1999). Interestingly, estradiol, but not progeserone, has consistently been linked to depression (Payne, 2003; Studd and Panay, 2004; Douma et al., 2005). Clearly further research is needed to clarify the combined role of these two streroid hormones on PPD.

In animal models of depression, support for the involvement of estrogen on depressive symptoms comes from studies examining the effects of ovariectomy and/or hormone replacement on behavioural tests for depression (Rachman et al., 1998; Bekku and Yoshimura, 2005). The Porsolt Forced Swim Test (FST) a measure of antidepressant efficacy (Porsolt et al, 1977; Lucki, 1997; Cryan et al., 2005) has been used as a measure of 'depressive' symptoms in animals (Galea et al., 2001; Dalla et al., 2004). This test involves placing an animal in a chamber filled with water (to a height such that the animals legs and tail cannot reach the bottom of the chamber) and measuring the amount of swimming, struggling, and immobility (Porsolt et al, 1977). Animal models of depression produce increased immobility and decreased active behaviours on these tests relative to control animals (Galea et al., 2001; Dalla et al., 2004), and clinically effective antidepressants have been shown to reduce the expression of immobility and increase the active behaviours (swimming, struggling), supporting the validity of the measure (Cryan et al., 2005). Rodent models of depression have demonstrated significant increases in immobility after ovariectomy compared to sham controls (Okada et al., 1997; Rachman et al., 1998; Frye and Wawrzycki, 2003; Dalla et al., 2004), and this effect can be attenuated with acute or chronic estrogen replacement, as well as by administering SSRI antidepressants (Rachman et al., 1998; Frye and Wawrzycki, 2003; Walf et al., 2004; Rocha et al., 2005).

Recent work has begun to address the role of steroid hormones on PPD. Work from our laboratory and others has recently employed a model which simulates the cycle of estradiol and progesterone observed during rodent pregnancy, commonly known as hormone simulated pregnancy (HSP; Rosenblatt et al., 1988). In our model, ovariectomized animals undergo a treatment regime where rats receive increasing doses of estradiol and progesterone for 23 days (the duration of normal gestation), after which hormones are abruptly withdrawn to mimic the postpartum period. Four days after the abrupt drop, during the 'postpartum' period, animals show increased immobility in the forced swim test, a behaviour which can be prevented by continuing treatment with estradiol (Galea et al., 2001; Stoffel and Craft, 2004). Intriguingly, despite these increased depressive symptoms in the 'postpartum' period, animals in this paradigm show no alterations in anxiety behaviours (as measured using the elevated plus maze) or general locomotion (Galea et al., 2001; Stoffel and Craft, 2004). This complements existing human studies of PPD and estrogen, where estrogen withdrawal may precipitate depressive symptoms in vulnerable women (Bloch et al, 2000). In addition, in our animal model of estradiol induced PPD we have shown that estradiol treatment after "estradiol withdrawal" alleviated the 'depressive' behavior shown in the forced swim test (Galea et al, 2001). This complements clinical research demonstrating that depressive symptoms during the postpartum may be alleviated (at least in part) by treatment with estrogen (Sichel et al., 1995; Gregoire et al., 1996; Ahokas et al., 2001).

We have recently investigated the role of adult hippocampal neurogenesis in our 'estradiol-withdrawal' model of PPD. Evidence from our laboratory indicates that the 'estradiol-withdrawal' model of PPD suppressed levels of hippocampal neurogenesis, via cell proliferation in adult female rats. Estradiol treatment, which alleviates the 'depressive' behaviour shown in the forced swim test, did not eliminate PPD-induced suppression of neurogenesis at least 24 h after injection with bromodeoxyuridine (Figure 1), suggesting that estradiol was not effective in treating this potential neural marker of depression. This compliments the work of Jayatissa et al (2006) who found that hippocampal cytogenesis was reduced in an animal model of depression. Interestingly in their model, antidepressants upregulated hippocampal cytogenesis to the same degree as controls but only in a subset of animals that also exhibited recovered depressive behaviour. These findings indicate that hippocampal cytogenesis was closely tied to the behavioral expression of depression. On going research in our laboratory is investigating the link between estradiol, antidepressants and hippocampal neurogenesis in our 'estradiol withdrawal' model of PPD.

While a growing body of evidence suggests that 'estradiol withdrawal' plays a key role in the development of PPD, the underlying mechanisms remain poorly understood. Current research in our laboratory is investigating the mechanism behind the role of estrogen in PPD with focus on the serotonergic system and growth factors. Estrogen has shown to influence the development of depressive symptoms through its agonistic interactions with the serotonergic system (Backstrom et al., 2003; Birzniece et al., 2005). Furthermore as stated earlier, Dalla et al (2004) report that estradiol-deficit female mice (ArKO) show more depressive systems than wildtype mice and these effects may be due to the organizational role of estradiol on the hippocampus serotonergic system. In addition estrogen has also been shown to play an important role in the regulation of brain-derived neurotrophic factor (BDNF) levels (reviewed in Scharfman and Maclusky, 2005), and research has demonstrated a role for BDNF in major depression (Eisch et al., 2003; Saarelainen et al., 2003; Koponen et al., 2005; Karege et al, 2002; Shimizu et al, 2003; Neumeister et al, 2005; Lommatzsch et al., 2006) and PPD (Lommatzsch et al., 2006). Intriguingly women with maternal depression have higher levels of cortisol than controls and BDNF levels are reduced during the perinatal period, which may contribute to PPD (Lommatzsch et al., 2006). Thus the abrupt loss of estradiol could trigger depressive symptoms through its effects on serotonin and/or BDNF.

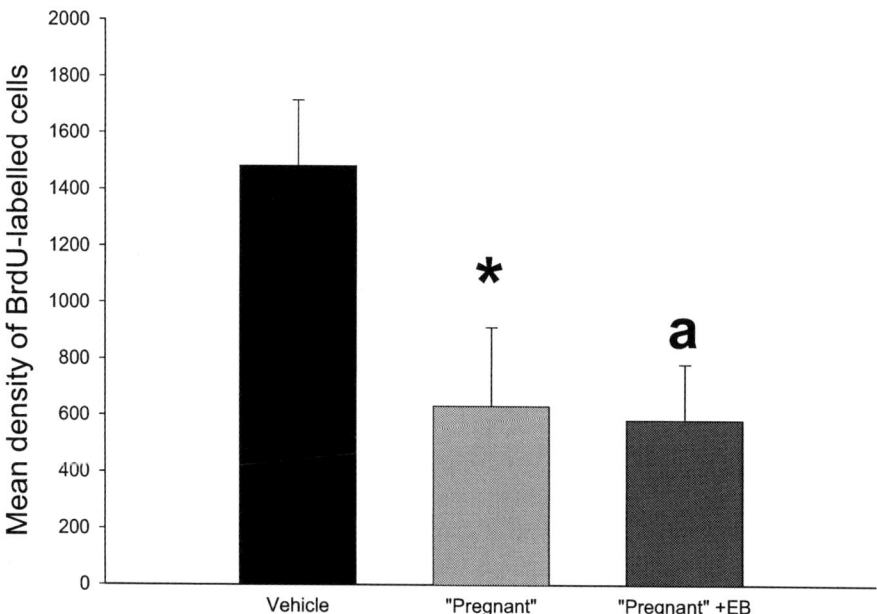

Figure 1. Mean density ($\pm$ SEM) of BrdU-labelled cells in the granule cell layer of the dentate gyrus of adult female rats. Fifteen ovariectomised Sprague-Dawley rats were placed into one of 3 groups: Vehicle, "Pregnant" and "Pregnant" + EB. Rats receive the same combination of estradiol and progesterone or oil injections s.c. as in Galea et al., 2001. On the 25th day, rats also received an i.p.injection of the cell synthesis marker bromodeoxyuridine (BrdU; 200 mg/kg) to label dividing cells and were perfused 24 hours later to examine cell proliferation. The "Pregnant" had significantly fewer proliferating cells than the vehicle group (p<.03), while there was a strong trend for the "Pregnant+EB" group to have fewer proliferating cells compared to the vehicle group (p<.06) 24 h after BrdU injection. Ormerod, Lieblich, Wide, Galea, personal communication.

It is important to note that this hypogonadal state during the postpartum does not occur in isolation. Pregnancy and the postpartum period are accompanied by an array of hormonal and physiological changes; including alterations to other hormones such as progesterone, oxytocin, and cortisol (Hendrick et al., 1998; Parry et al., 2003; Spinelli, 2005; Driscoll, 2006). Furthermore, while estrogen treatment may be an important method of treating PPD, it only appears to alleviate depressive symptoms in a subset of patients (reviewed in Karuppaswamy and Vlies, 2003). It is likely that, while estrogen withdrawal may precipitate depressive symptoms in predisposed women, a collection of other genetic and environmental factors will contribute to this underlying vulnerability (Payne, 2003; Studd and Panay, 2004; Strous et al., 2006). The "estrogen withdrawal" model of PPD allows for an important framework within which to examine these different underlying mechanisms and predisposition, and, through convergence with clinical trials, may greatly improve our understanding of the mechanism and treatment of postpartum depression.

ii. The Role of Corticosterone in an Animal Model of PPD

As mentioned earlier, the stress of pregnancy and motherhood has been shown to contribute to postpartum depression (O'Hara et al., 1991; O'Hara and Swain, 1996; Bernazzani et al, 1997; Beck 2001; Misdrahi et al., 2005) and may be associated with abnormal HPA axis funtioning at this time (Carter et al, 2001; Magiakou et al., 1996). This is interesting as depression is often associated with hypercortisolism and an abnormal hypothalamic-pituitary-adrenal (HPA) axis function in humans (Mackin and Young, 2004; Newport et al., 2002a; Parker et al., 2003). In fact, sustained elevated glucocorticoid levels, as seen after chronic stress, may be neurotoxic and a major risk factor for the development of depressive symptoms (Mackin and Young, 2004). In addition, gestational stress has been shown to induce postpartum depression-like behaviour in the mother, alter maternal care, and have deleterious effects on the offspring (Smith et al., 2004; Tu et al., 2005; Newport et al., 2002b). Thus exposure to chronic stress and/or high levels of cortisol/corticosterone during the postpartum may be a major contributing factor for PPD and have a deleterious effect on the brain and behaviour of offspring.

Recently, corticosterone has been shown to play a role in the modulation of ongoing maternal behaviors (Rees et al., 2004; Graham et al, 2005). High levels of cortisol have been negatively correlated with maternal care in primates (Bahr et al., 1998; Bardi et al., 2003). Bahr et al (1998) found that the time a mother spent with her infant decreased as maternal stress, indicated by high cortisol, increased. Bardi et al (2003) found that postpartum cortisol levels also showed a significant positive association with the rate of infant rejection in Japanese Macaques. In addition, depressed human mothers are less positive towards their infants (Field, 1998), touch their infants less (Ferber, 2004) and are more likely to exhibit higher levels of cortisol (Lommatzsch et al., 2005). However, in new mothers that are not depressed, studies suggest that cortisol levels are positively correlated with attractiveness to infant odor (Fleming et al., 1987; Fleming et al., 1997). With regards to offspring, a moderate elevation of corticosterone in lactating dams leads to a "beneficial" outcome in the offspring with increased hippocampal corticosteroid receptors, improved learning and memory

(Casolini et al., 1997; Catalani et al., 2000; Catalani et al., 2002), long-lasting changes in the hippocampal CA1 synaptic plasticity (Domenici et al., 1996), and better "coping" with stressful situations throughout their life (Catalani et al., 2000). These findings indicate that although glucocorticoids are needed for normal maternal care, higher levels of corticosterone may lead to decreased maternal care, and/or depressive symptoms in offspring. Therefore, we developed a model of PPD to examine the role of elevated levels of corticosterone during the post partum on depressive-like behavior in the dams and resulting effects on changes in offspring brain and behaviour.

In our corticosterone model of PPD, we found that administration of high levels of corticosterone to dams during the postpartum resulted in significant depressive-like behaviour in the dams (Figure 2), as measured by the forced swim test, and alterations in the amount of nursing and licking behavior elicited by the dam (Brummelte et al., 2006). In addition, we found a decrease in postnatal hippocampal neurogenesis in male, but not female, offspring from the CORT-treated dams as well as higher levels of anxiety, activity levels, and aggression in offspring of CORT-treated dams (Brummelte et al., 2006) (Figure 3). This corticosterone-induced model of PPD allows for the examination of the role of corticosterone on the brain and behaviour of mothers and her offspring which will not only improve our understanding of mechanism of PPD in the mother, but also effects on her children. Future work aims to further investigate neural and behavioural effects of elevated corticosterone and chronic stress on the etiology of PPD and its effect on offspring development.

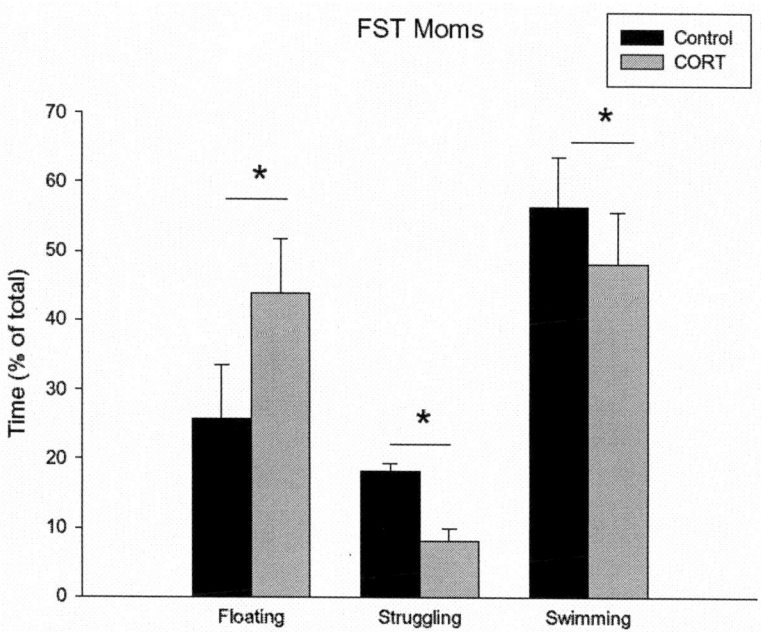

Figure 2. Mean (± SEM) percent of time spent floating, struggling or swimming in control and CORT dams in the Porsolt Forced Swim Test. Sprague-Dawley dams were treated with either CORT (40mg/kg) or sesame oil injections daily for 26 days beginning the day after giving birth. Dams were tested in the Forced Swim Test on Days 24-26 postpartum. CORT dams exhibit a 'depressive-like' behavior with less struggling and greater immobility than control dams (p≤ .017). Taken from Brummelte et al., 2006.

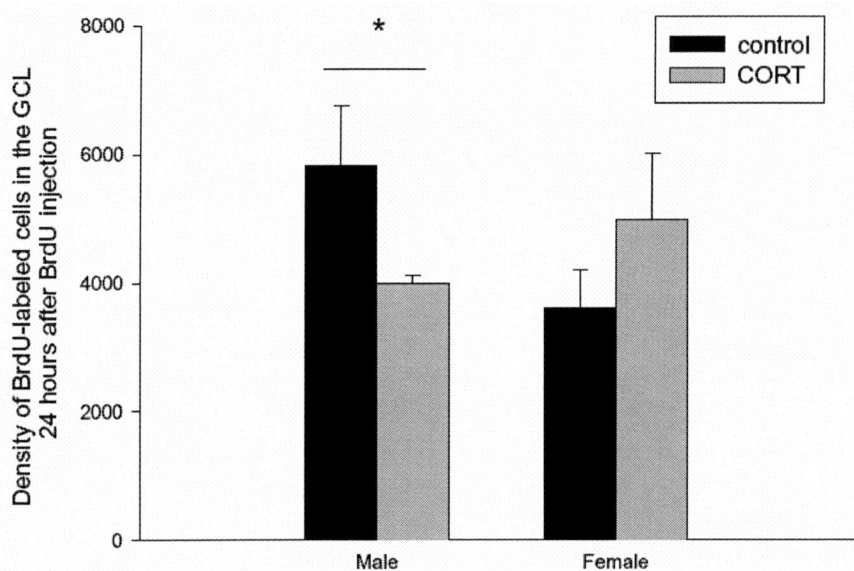

Figure 3. Mean density (± SEM) of BrdU-labeled cells in the granule cell layer (GCL) of males and female offspring of control- and CORT-treated dams at 21 days of age. Sprague-Dawley dams were treated with either CORT (40mg/kg) or sesame oil injections daily for 26 days beginning the day after giving birth. To investigate the effects of treatment on hippocampal postnatal cell proliferation in the offspring, males and females from treated dams were injected with BrdU (50mg/kg) on postnatal day 21 and perfused 24 hours. Male pups from CORT dams had significantly lower levels of cell proliferation in the GCL than males from control dams ($p \leq .007$). Taken from Brummelte et al., 2006.

iii. The Possible Role of other Steroid Hormones on PPD

Although the effects of progesterone on the development of PPD has yet to be determined, animal models of depression have demonstrated that progesterone may play a role in alleviating depressive symptoms (Bernardi et al., 1989; Martinez-Mota et al., 1999). Bernardi et al (1989) found that treatment with both estradiol and progesterone alleviated 'depressive' behavior in ovariectomised rats and Martinez-Mota et al (1999) found that treatment with progesterone alone reduced 'depressive' behavior in ovariectomised rats without modifying locomotor activity. Interestingly, our 'estradiol withdrawal' model of PPD also involves withdrawal of progesterone, although to a lesser extent (Galea et al, 2001). This suggests that although estradiol may alleviate 'depressive' behaviors in this model (Galea et al., 2001), perhaps both estradiol and progesterone are needed to alleviate the suppression seen in adult hippocamal neurogenesis (Ormerod, Lieblich, Wide and Galea, personal communication).

The neuroactive metabolites and precursors of progesterone may also be significant contributors to PPD. These neurosteroids are mainly synthesized de novo from cholesterol in the central nervous system, partly independent of peripheral steroidogenic endocrine glands (Stoffel-Wagner, 2001). In particular, cholesterol is converted to pregnanolone, which is further metabolized to pregnanes and androstanes. Of possible importance to the neurobiological etiology of depression and PPD are the pregnanes, 3α, 5αtetrahydoprogesterone (allopregnanolone) and 3α, 5α-tetrahydrodeoxycorticosterone (3α, 5α-THDOC), and the androstane dehydroepiandrosterone (DHEA) (van Broekhoven and Verkes, 2003; Zonana and Gorman, 2005).

Allopregnanolone, a neuroactive metabolite of progesterone, may be a significant contributor to PPD (Nappi et al., 2001; reviewed in Herbison, 2001). This steroid is commonly considered a neurosteroid and is mainly synthesized de novo from cholesterol in the central nervous system, but the majority of allopregnanolone in the brain is derived from circulating progesterone (Corpechor et al., 1993; reviewed in Herbison, 2001). Allopregnanolone has been found to play a role in etiology of depression (van Broekhoven and Verkes, 2003; Zonana and Gorman, 2005) and may also contribute to mood changes during the postpartum (Nappi et al., 2001). In depressed patients, allopregnanolone levels are low (Uzunova et al, 1998; Romeo et al, 1998; Strohle et al., 1999), but are normalised after effective treatment with antidepressants (Uzunova et al., 1998; Romeo et al., 1998). In a rodent model of depression, administration of allopregnanolone resulted in antidepressive effects as measured by the forced swim test (Khisti et al., 2000). As well, studies in rats have shown an allopregnanolone-induced decrease in corticotrophin-releasing hormone (CRH) and therefore possibly result in a reduction in anxiety and/or stress reactivity produced by increased CRH (Patchev et al., 1996). In addition, Nappi et al (2001) have found that allopregnanolone levels are significantly decreased in women reporting postpartum blues. These lines of research suggest a major role for allopregnanolone in the pathophysiology of post partum depression.

Both allopregnanolone and 3α, 5α- THDOC are positive allosteric modulators of the GABA-A receptor, therefore it would be expected that the plasma levels of these two neurosteroids would follow a similar pattern during depression, however, this is not the case: Strohle et al (2000) found that depressed patients have higher plasma levels of 3α, 5α-THDOC than controls, which is opposite to what was reported for allopregnanolone (Uzunova et al, 1998; Romeo et al, 1998; Strohle et al., 1999). Interestingly, 3α, 5α- THDOC levels were not found to be significantly influenced by antidepressant treatment (Strohle et al., 2000).

DHEA is a neurosteroid that increases during the first and second trimester and decreases after parturition for 11 months postpartum (Tagawa et al., 2004). It also has been shown to play a role in depression and may also be a modulator of PPD. Oral administration of DHEA decreased depressive symptoms in patients with major depression (Broekhoven and Verkes, 2003). In animals, administration of DHEA in models of depression resulted in antidepressive effects as measured by the forced swim test (Urani et al. 2001). In addition, estradiol withdrawal in female rats has been shown to increase corticol levels of DHEA-S (the sulfate derivative of DHEA) (Maayan et al, 2005).

Further research should aim to determine the role of progesterone, its precursors and metabolites, in animal models of PPD as well as the interaction of these steroids with other hormones and systems, such as corticosterone and the HPA axis.

iv. Conclusions

PPD is a debilitating disease that affects 11% of mothers and, in turn, their children. In order to understand the etiology and treatment of this disease research has aimed to study the role of fluctuating levels of steroid hormones in the onset of this disorder. We have developed two animal models of PPD to evaluate the neural and behavioral effects of 1) estradiol-withdrawal after parturition in the mother, and 2) elevated corticosterone during the postpartum in the mother and offspring. These models have provided insight into the effects of these steroid hormones on the brain and behaviour of the mother and the offspring. Future work aims to increase our knowledge of PPD through the development of these and other animal models. Understanding the etiology and treatment of this disorder is essential for determining how we can promote well-being in mothers and their children.

ACKNOWLEDGEMENTS

We would like to thank Dr. Brandi Ormerod, Susie Brummelte, Lucille Hoover, Stephanie Lieblich, and Jen Wide for their contributions to this research. This work was funded by a Human Early Learning Program (HELP) grant, a National Alliance for Research on Schizophrenia and Depression (NARSAD) Award to LAMG. The researchers gratefully acknowledge funding from the BC Ministry of Children and Family Development through the Human Early Learning Partnership. The views presented here are solely those of the authors and do not represent the policy of HELP or the Province. JLP holds a Michael Smith Senior Graduate Award. CB holds a NSERC graduate award. LAMG is a Michael Smith Senior Scholar.

REFERENCES

Ahokas, A.. Kaukoranta, J., Wahlbeck, K., Aito, M. (2001). Estrogen deficiency in severe postpartum depression: successful treatment with sublingual physiologic 17beta-estradiol: a preliminary study. *J Clin Psychiatry, 62*, 332-336.

Altshuler, L. L., Hendrick, V., & Cohen, L. S. (2000). An Update on Mood and Anxiety Disorders During Pregnancy and the Postpartum Period. Prim.Care Companion. *J.Clin.Psychiatry, 2*, 217-222.

Backstrom, T., Andersson, A., Andree, L., Birzniece, V., Bixo, M., Bjorn, I., Haage, D., Isaksson, M., Johansson, I.M., Lindblad, C., Lundgren, P., Nyberg, S., Odmark, I. S., Stromberg, J., Sundstrom-Poromaa, I., Turkmen, S., Wahlstrom, G., Wang, M., Wihlback, A. C., Zhu, D., & Zingmark, E. (2003). Pathogenesis in menstrual cycle-linked CNS disorders. *Ann N Y Acad Sci, 1007*, 42-53.

Bahr, N. I., Pryce, C. R., Dobeli, M., & Martin, R. D. (1998). Evidence from urinary cortisol that maternal behavior is related to stress in gorillas. *Physiol Behav., 64*, 429-437.

Bardi, M., Shimizu, K., Barrett, G. M., Borgognini-Tarli, S. M., & Huffman, M. A. (2003). Peripartum cortisol levels and mother-infant interactions in Japanese macaques. *Am.J.Phys.Anthropol., 120*, 298-304.

Beck, C. T. (2001). Predictors of postpartum depression: an update. *Nursing Research, 50*, 275-85.

Bekku, N., & Yoshimura, H. (2005). Animal model of menopausal depressive-like state in female mice: prolongation of immobility time in the forced swimming test following ovariectomy. *Psychopharmacology (Berl), 183*, 300-307.

Bernardi, M., Vergoni, A.V., Sandrini, M. & Tagliavini, S. B. (1989). Influence of ovariectormy, estradiol and progesterone on the/behavior of mice in an experimental model of depression. *Physiol Behav, 45*, 1067–1068.

Bernazzani, O., Saucier, J. F., David, H., & Borgeat, F. (1997). Psychosocial predictors of depressive symptomatology level in postpartum women. *J Affect Disord, 46*, 39-49.

Birzniece, V., Backstrom, T., Johansson, I. M., Lindblad, C., Lundgren, P., Lofgren, M., Olsson, T., Ragagnin, G., Taube, M., Turkmen, S., Wahlstrom, G., Wang, M. D., Wihlback, A. C., & Zhu, D. (2005). Neuroactive steroid effects on cognitive functions with a focus on the serotonin and GABA systems. *Brain Res Brain Res Rev*, Epub ahead of print.

Bloch, M., Daly, R. C., & Rubinow, D. R. (2003). Endocrine factors in the etiology of postpartum depression. *Compr.Psychiatry, 44*, 234-246

Bloch M., Rubinow, D.R., Schmidt, P.J., Lotsikas, A., Chrousos, G.P., & Cizza, G. (2005) Cortisol response to ovine corticotropin-releasing hormone in a model of pregnancy and parturition in euthymic women with and without a history of postpartum depression. *J Clin Endocrinol Metab, 90*, 695-699.

Bloch, M., Schmidt, P. J., Danaceau, M., Murphy, J., Nieman, L., & Rubinow, D. R. (2000). Effects of gonadal steroids in women with a history of postpartum depression. *Am J Psychiatry, 157*, 924-930.

Boulware, M. I., & Mermelstein, P.G. (2005). The influence of estradiol on nervous system function. *Drug News Perspect, 18*, 631-637.

Brummelte, S., Pawluski, J. L., & Galea, L. A. (2006). High postpartum levels of corticosterone given to dams influence postnatal neurogenesis and behaviour of offspring: A possible model of post-partum depression. *Hormones and Behavior, 50*, 372-380.

Buckwalter, J. G., Stanczyk, F. Z., McCleary, C. A., et al. (1999). Pregnancy the postpartum, and steroid hormones: effects on cognition and mood. *Psychoneuroendocrinology, 24*, 69-84.

Campbell, S., & Macqueen, G. (2004). The role of the hippocampus in the pathophysiology of major depression. *J Psychiatry Neurosci, 29*, 417-426.

Campbell, S., Marriott, M., Nahmias, C., & MacQueen, G. M. (2004). Lower hippocampal volume in patients suffering from depression: a meta-analysis. *Am J Psychiatry, 161*, 598-607.

Carter, C. S., Altemus, M., Chrousos, G. P. (2001). Neuroendocrine and emotional changes in the post-partum period. *Prog Brain Res., 133*, 241-9.

Casolini, P., Cigliana, G., Alema, G. S., Ruggieri, V., Angelucci, L., & Catalani, A. (1997). Effect of increased maternal corticosterone during lactation on hippocampal corticosteroid receptors, stress response and learning in offspring in the early stages of life. *Neuroscience, 79*, 1005-1012.

Catalani, A., Casolini, P., Cigliana, G., Scaccianoce, S., Consoli, C., Cinque, C., Zuena, A. R., & Angelucci, L., (2002). Maternal corticosterone influences behavior, stress response and corticosteroid receptors in the female rat. *Pharmacol.Biochem.Behav., 73*, 105-114.

Catalani, A., Casolini, P., Scaccianoce, S., Patacchioli, F. R., Spinozzi, P., & Angelucci, L. (2000). Maternal corticosterone during lactation permanently affects brain corticosteroid receptors, stress response and behaviour in rat progeny. *Neuroscience, 100*, 319-325.

Cooper, P. J., & Murray, L. (1995). Course and recurrence of postnatal depression. Evidence for the specificity of the diagnostic concept. *Br J Psychiatry, 166*, 191-195.

Cryan, J. F., Valentino, R. J., & Lucki, I. (2005). Assessing substrates underlying the behavioral effects of antidepressants using the modified rat forced swimming test. *Neurosci Biobehav Rev, 29*, 547-569.

Dalla, C., Antoniou, K., Papadopoulou-Daifoti, Z., Balthazart. J,, Bakker, J. (2004). Oestrogen-deficient female aromatase knockout (ArKO) mice exhibit depressive-like symptomatology. *Eur J Neurosci, 20*, 217-228.

De Kloet, E. R. (2004). Hormones and the stressed brain. *Ann N Y Acad Sci., 1018*, 1-15.

Domenici, M. R., Casolini, P., Catalani, A., Ruggieri, V., Angelucci, L., & Sagratella, S. (1996). Reduced hippocampal in vitro CA1 long-term potentiation in rat offsprings with increased circulating corticosterone during neonatal life. *Neurosci.Lett., 218*, 72-74.

Douma, S. L., Husband, C., O'Donnell, M. E., Barwin, B. N., Woodend, A. K. (2005). Estrogen-related mood disorders: reproductive life cycle factors. *ANS Adv Nurs Sci, 28*, 364-375.

Driscoll, J. W. (2006). Postpartum depression: the state of the science. *J Perinat Neonatal Nurs, 20*, 40-42.

Eisch, A. J., Bolanos, C.A., de Wit, J., Simonak, R.D., Pudiak, C.M., Barrot, M., Verhaagen, J., & Nestler, E.J. (2003). Brain-derived neurotrophic factor in the ventral midbrain-nucleus accumbens pathway: a role in depression. *Biol Psychiatry, 54*, 994-1005.

Feksi, A., Harris, B., Walker, R. F., Riad-Fahmy, D., & Newcombe, R. G. (1984). 'Maternity blues' and hormone levels in saliva. *J Affect Disord, 6*, 351-355.

Ferber, S.G. (2004). The nature of touch in mothers experiencing maternity blues: the contribution of parity. *Early Hum.Dev,. 79*, 65-75.

Field, T., (1998). Maternal depression effects on infants and early interventions. *Prev.Med., 27*, 200-203.

Fleming, A. S., Steiner, M., & Anderson, V. (1987). Hormonal and attitudinal correlates of maternal behavior during the early postpartum period in first-time mothers. *J Reprod Inf Psychol, 5*, 193-205.

Fleming, A. S., Steiner, M., & Corter, C. (1997). Cortisol, hedonics, and maternal responsiveness in human mothers. *Horm.Behav, 32*, 85-98.

Frye, C. A., & Wawrzycki, J. (2003). Effect of prenatal stress and gonadal hormone condition on depressive behaviors of female and male rats. *Horm Behav, 44*, 319-326.

Galea, L. A, Wide, J. K., Barr, A. M. (2001). Estradiol alleviates depressive-like symptoms in a novel animal model of post-partum depression. *Behav Brain Res, 122*, 1-9.

Georgiopoulos, A. M., Bryan, T. L., Yawn, B. P., Houston, M. S., Rummans, T. A., & Therneau, T. M. (1999). Population-based screening for postpartum depression. *Obstet. Gynecol., 93*, 653-657.

Graham, M. D., Rees, S. L., Steiner, M., & Fleming, A. S. (2006). The effects of adrenalectomy and corticosterone replacement on maternal memory in postpartum rats. *Horm Behav., 49(3)*, 353-361.

Gregoire, A. J., Kumar, R., Everitt, B., Henderson, A. F., & Studd, J. W. (1996). Transdermal oestrogen for treatment of severe postnatal depression. *Lancet, 347*, 930-933.

Gregus, A., Wintink, A. J., Davis, A. C., & Kalynchuk, L. E. (2005). Effect of repeated corticosterone injections and restraint stress on anxiety and depression-like behavior in male rats. *Behav.Brain Res., 156*, 105-114.

Harris, B., Lovett, L., Smith, J., Read, G., Walker, R., & Newcombe, R. G. (1996). Cardiff puerperal mood and hormone study. III. Postnatal depression at 5 to 6 weeks postpartum, and its hormonal correlates across the peripartum period. *Br J Psychiatry, 168*, 739-744.

Heidrich, A., Schleyer, M., & Spingler, H., et al. (1994). Postpartum blues: relationship between not-protein bound steroid hormones in plasma and postpartum mood changes. *J Affect Disord, 30*, 93-98.

Hendrick, V., Altshuler, L.L., & Suri, R. (1998). Hormonal changes in the postpartum and implications for postpartum depression. *Psychosomatics, 39*, 93-101.

Herbison, A. E. (2001). Physiological roles for the neurosteroid allopregnanolone in the modulation of brain function during pregnancy and parturition. *Prog Brain Res., 133*, 39-47.

Huang, G. J., & Herbert, J. (2005). Serotonin modulates the suppressive effects of corticosterone on proliferating progenitor cells in the dentate gyrus of the hippocampus in the adult rat. *Neuropsychopharmacology, 30*, 231-241.

Jaako-Movits, K., & Zharkovsky, A. (2005). Impaired fear memory and decreased hippocampal neurogenesis following olfactory bulbectomy in rats. *Eur J Neurosci., 22*, 2871-2878.

Jayatissa, M. N., Bisgaard, C., Tingstrom, A., Papp, M., & Wiborg, O. (2006). Hippocampal Cytogenesis Correlates to Escitalopram-Mediated Recovery in a Chronic Mild Stress Rat Model of Depression. *Neuropsychopharmacology*. Epub ahead of print.

Kalynchuk, L. E., Gregus, A., Boudreau, D., & Perrot-Sinal, T. S. (2004). Corticosterone increases depression-like behavior, with some effects on predator odor-induced defensive behavior, in male and female rats. *Behav.Neurosci., 118*, 1365-1377.

Karuppaswamy, J., & Vlies, R. (2003). The benefit of oestrogens and progestogens in postnatal depression. *J Obstet Gynaecol., 23*, 341-346.

Karege, F., Perret, G., Bondolfi, G., Schwald, M., Bertschy, G., & Aubry, J.M. (2002). Decreased serum brain-derived neurotrophic factor levels in major depressed patients. *Psychiatry Res.,109*, 143-148.

Khisti, R. T., Chopde, C. T., & Jain, S. P. (2000). Antidepressant-like effect of the neurosteroid 3 alpha-hydroxy-5 alpha-pregnan-20-one in mice forced swim test. *Pharmacol Biochem Behav, 67*, 137–143.

Koponen, E., Rantamaki, T., Voikar, V., Saarelainen, T., MacDonald, E., & Castren, E. (2005). Enhanced BDNF signaling is associated with an antidepressant-like behavioral response and changes in brain monoamines. *Cell Mol Neurobiol, 25*, 973-980.

Kuevi, V., Causon, R., Dixson, AF., et al. (1983). Plasma amine and hormone changes in 'post-partum blues'. *Clin Endocrinol, 19*, 39-46.

Lehtinen, V., & Joukamaa, M. (1994). Epidemiology of depression: prevalence, risk factors and treatment situation. *Acta Psychiatr. Scand. Suppl., 377*, 7–10.

Lommatzsch, M., Hornych, K., Zingler, C., Schuff-Werner, P., Hoppner, J., & Virchow, J.C. (2006). Maternal serum concentrations of BDNF and depression in the perinatal period. *Psychoneuroendocrinology, 31*:388-394.

Lucki, I. (1997). The forced swimming test as a model for core and component behavioral effects of antidepressant drugs. *Behav.Pharmacol., 8*, 523-532.

Maayan, R., Strous, R. D., Abou-Kaoud, M., & Weizman, A. (2005). The effect of 17beta estradiol withdrawal on the level of brain and peripheral neurosteroids in ovarectomized rats. *Neurosci Lett., 384(1-2)*, 156-161.

Mackin, P., & Young, A. H. (2004). The Role of Cortisol and Depression: Exploring New Opportunities for Treatments. *Psychiatric Times, 21*, 92-95.

MacQueen, G. M., Campbell, S., McEwen, B. S., Macdonald, K., Amano, S., Joffe, R.T., Nahmias, C., & Young, L.T. (2003). Course of illness, hippocampal function, and hippocampal volume in major depression. *Proc Natl Acad Sci U S A, 100*, 1387-1392.

Magiakou, M. A., Mastorakos, G., Rabin, D., Dubbert, B., Gold, P.W., & Chrousos, G.P. (1996). Hypothalamic corticotropin-releasing hormone suppression during the postpartum period: implications for the increase in psychiatric manifestations at this time. *J Clin Endocrinol Metab., 81(5)*, 1912-1917.

Malberg, J. E., Eisch, A. J., Nestler, E. J., & Duman, R. S. (2000). Chronic antidepressant treatment increases neurogenesis in adult rat hippocampus. *J Neurosci, 20*, 9104-9110.

Martinez-Mota, L., Contreras, C. M., & Saavedra, M. (1999). Progesterone reduced immobility in rats forced to swim. *Arch. Med. Res, 30(4)*, 286–289.

McEwen, B. (2002). Estrogen actions throughout the brain. *Recent Prog Horm Res, 57*, 357-384.

Misdrahi, D., Pardon, M. C., Perez-Diaz, F., Hanoun, N., & Cohen-Salmon, C. (2005). Prepartum chronic ultramild stress increases corticosterone and estradiol levels in gestating mice: Implications for postpartum depressive disorders. *Psychiatry Res., 137*, 123-130.

Murray, L., & Cooper, P. (1997). Effects of postnatal depression on infant development. *Arch.Dis.Child, 77*, 99-101.

Nappi, R. E., Petraglia, F., Luisi, S., Polatti, F., Farina, C., & Genazzani, A.R. (2001). Serum allopregnanolone in women with postpartum 'blues'. *Obstet Gynecol, 97*, 77–80.

Newport, D. J., Stowe, Z. N., & Nemeroff, C. B. (2002a). Parental depression: animal models of an adverse life event. *Am.J.Psychiatry, 159*, 1265-1283.

Newport, D. J., Wilcox, M. M., & Stowe, Z. N. (2002b). Maternal depression: a child's first adverse life event. *Semin.Clin.Neuropsychiatry, 7*, 113-119.

Neumeister, A., Yuan, P., Young, T. A., Bonne, O., Luckenbaugh, D. A., Charney, D. S., & Manji, H. (2005). Effects of tryptophan depletion on serum levels of brain-derived neurotrophic factor in unmedicated patients with remitted depression and healthy subjects. *Am J Psychiatry, 162*, 805-807.

Nomura, Y., Wickramaratne, P. J., Warner, V., Mufson, L., & Weissman, M. M. (2002). Family discord, parental depression, and psychopathology in offspring: ten-year follow-up. *J.Am.Acad.Child Adolesc.Psychiatry, 41*, 402-409.

Nott, P. N., Franklin, M., Armitage, C., & Gelder, M. G. (1976). Hormonal changes and mood in the puerperium. *Br J Psychiatry, 128*, 379-383.

O'Hara, M. W., & Swain, A. M. (1996). Rates and risk of postpartum depression-a meta-analysis. *Int Rev Psychiatry, 8*, 37-54.

O'Hara, M.W., Schlechte, J. A., Lewis, D.A., & Varner, M. W. (1991). Controlled prospective study of postpartum mood disorders: Psychological, environmental, and hormonal variables. *J Abnorm Psychol, 100*, 63-73.

Okada, M., Hayashi, N., Kometani, M., Nakao, K., & Inukai, T. (1997). Influences of ovariectomy and continuous replacement of 17beta-estradiol on the tail skin temperature and behavior in the forced swimming test in rats. *Jpn J Pharmacol, 73*, 93-96.

Parry, B. L., Sorenson, D. L., Meliska, C. J., Basavaraj, N., Zirpoli, G. G., Gamst, A., & Hauger, R. (2003). Hormonal basis of mood and postpartum disorders. *Curr Womens Health Rep, 3*, 230-235.

Parker, K. J., Schatzberg, A. F., & Lyons, D. M. (2003). Neuroendocrine aspects of hypercortisolism in major depression. *Horm.Behav., 43*, 60-66.

Patchev, V. K., Hassan, A. H., Holsboer, D. F., & Almeida, O. F. (1996). The neurosteroid tetrahydroprogesterone attenuates the endocrine response to stress and exerts glucocorticoid-like effects on vasopressin gene transcription in the rat hypothalamus. *Neuropsychopharmacology, 15*, 533–540.

Payne, J. L. (2003). The role of estrogen in mood disorders in women. *Int Rev Psychiatry, 15*, 280-290.

Perez, A., Vela, P., Masnick, G. S., & Potter, R. G. (1972). First ovulation after childbirth: the effect of breast-feeding. *Am J Obstet Gynecol, 114*, 1041-1047.

Pham, K., Nacher, J., Hof, P. R., & McEwen, B. S. (2003). Repeated restraint stress suppresses neurogenesis and induces biphasic PSA-NCAM expression in the adult rat dentate gyrus. *Eur.J Neurosci, 17*, 879-886.

Porsolt, R. D., LePichon, M., Jalfre, M. (1977). Depression: a new animal model sensitive to antidepressant treatments. *Nature, 266*, 730-732.

Rachman, I. M., Unnerstall, J. R., Pfaff, D. W., & Cohen, R. S. (1998). Estrogen alters behavior and forebrain c-fos expression in ovariectomized rats subjected to the forced swim test. *Proc Natl Acad Sci U S A, 95*, 13941-13946.

Rees, S. L., Panesar, S., Steiner, M., & Fleming, A. S. (2004). The effects of adrenalectomy and corticosterone replacement on maternal behavior in the postpartum rat. *Horm.Behav., 46*, 411-419.

Righetti, P. L., Dell'Avanzo, M., Grigio, M., & Nicolini, U. (2005). Maternal/paternal antenatal attachment and fourth-dimensional ultrasound technique: a preliminary report. *Br.J Psychol, 96*, 129-137.

Rocha, B. A., Fleischer, R., Schaeffer, J. M., Rohrer, S. P., & Hickey, G. J. (2005). 17 Beta-estradiol-induced antidepressant-like effect in the forced swim test is absent in estrogen receptor-beta knockout (BERKO) mice. *Psychopharmacology (Berl), 179*, 637-643.

Romeo, E., Strohle, A., Spalletta, G., di Michele, F., Hermann, B., Holsboer, F., Pasini, A., & Rupprecht, R. (1998). Effects of antidepressant treatment on neuroactive steroids in major depression. *Am J Psychiatry*, 1998, 155:910–913.

Rosenblatt, J. S., Mayer, A. D., & Giordano A. L. (1988). Hormonal basis during pregnancy for the onset of maternal behavior in the rat. *Psychoneuroendocrinolgy, 13*, 29–42.

Saarelainen, T., Hendolin, P., Lucas, G., Koponen, E., Sairanen, M., MacDonald, E., Agerman, K., Haapasalo, A., Nawa, H., Aloyz, R., Ernfors, P., & Castren, E. (2003). Activation of the TrkB neurotrophin receptor is induced by antidepressant drugs and is required for antidepressant-induced behavioral effects. *J Neurosci, 23*, 349-357.

Santarelli, L., Saxe, M., Gross, C., Surget, A., Battaglia, F., Dulawa, S., Weisstaub, N., Lee, J., Duman, R., Arancio, O., Belzung, C., & Hen, R. (2003). Requirement of hippocampal neurogenesis for the behavioral effects of antidepressants. *Science, 301*, 805-809.

Scharfman, H. E., & Maclusky, N. J. (2005). Similarities between actions of estrogen and BDNF in the hippocampus: coincidence or clue? *Trends Neurosci, 28*, 79-85.

Sheline, Y. I., Sanghavi, M., Mintun, M. A., & Gado, M. H. (1999). Depression duration but not age predicts hippocampal volume loss in medically healthy women with recurrent major depression. *J Neurosci, 19*, 5034-5043.

Shimizu, E., Hashimoto, K., Okamura, N., Koike, K., Komatsu, N., Kumakiri, C., Nakazato, M., Watanabe, H., Shinoda, N., Okada, S., & Iyo, M. (2003). Alterations of serum levels of brain-derived neurotrophic factor (BDNF) in depressed patients with or without antidepressants. *Biol Psychiatry, 54*, 70-75.

Shively, C. A., Laber-Laird, K., Anton, R. F. (1997). Behavior and physiology of social stress and depression in female cynomolgus monkeys. *Biol Psychiatry., 41(8)*, 871-82.

Sichel, D. A., Cohen, L. S., Robertson, L. M., Ruttenberg, A., & Rosenbaum, J. F. (1995). Prophylactic estrogen in recurrent postpartum affective disorder. *Biol Psychiatry, 38*, 814-818.

Smith, J. W., Seckl, J. R., Evans, A. T., Costall, B., & Smythe, J. W. (2004). Gestational stress induces post-partum depression-like behaviour and alters maternal care in rats. *Psychoneuroendocrinology, 29*, 227-244.

Smith, S. S., Gong, Q. H., Hsu, F. C., Markowitz, R. S., French-Mullen, J. M. H., & Li, X. (1998). GABAA receptor alpha-4 subunit suppression prevents withdrawal properties of an endogenous steroid. *Nature, 392*, 926-930.

Soldin, O. P., Guo, T., Weiderpass, E., Tractenberg, R. E., Hilakivi-Clarke, L., & Soldin, S. J. (2005). Steroid hormone levels in pregnancy and 1 year postpartum using isotope dilution tandem mass spectrometry. *Fertil Steril., 84(3)*, 701-710.

Spinelli, M. G. (2005). Neuroendocrine effects on mood. *Rev Endocr Metab Disord, 6*, 109-115.

Steiner, M., Dunn, E., & Born, L. (2003). Hormones and mood: from menarche to menopause and beyond. *J Affect Disord, 74*, 67-83.

Stoffel, E. C., & Craft, R. M. (2004). Ovarian hormone withdrawal-induced "depression" in female rats. *Physiol Behav, 83*, 505-513.

Stoffel-Wagner, B. (2001). Neurosteroid metabolism in the human brain. *Eur J Endocrinol, 145*, 669–679.

Strohle, A., Pasini, A., Romeo, E., Hermann, B., Spalletta, G., di Michele, F., Holsboer, F., & Rupprecht, R. (2000). Fluoxetine decreases concentrations of 3 alpha, 5 alpha tetrahydrodeoxycorticosterone (THDOC) in major depression. *J Psychiatr Res, 34*, 183–186.

Strohle, A., Romeo, E., Hermann, B., Pasini, A., Spalletta, G., diMichele, F., Holsboer, F., Rupprecht, R. (1999). Concentrations of 3α reduced neuroactive steroids and their precursors in plasma of patients with major depression and after clinical recovery. *Biol Psychiatry, 45*, 274–277.

Strous, R. D., Maayan, R., & Weizman, A. (2006). The relevance of neurosteroids to clinical psychiatry: From the laboratory to the bedside. *Eur Neuropsychopharmacol, 16*, 155-169.

Studd, J., & Panay, N. (2004). Hormones and depression in women. *Climacteric, 7*, 338-346.

Swaab, D. F., Bao, A. M., & Lucassen, P. J. (2005). The stress system in the human brain in depression and neurodegeneration. *Ageing Res Rev, 4*, 141-194.

Tu, M. T., Lupien, S. J., & Walker, C. D. (2005). Measuring stress responses in postpartum mothers: perspectives from studies in human and animal populations. *Stress. 8*, 19-34.

Urani, A., Roman, F. J., Phan, V. L., Su, T. P., & Maurice, T. (2001). The antidepressant-like effect induced by sigma(1)-receptor agonists and neuroactive steroids in mice submitted to the forced swimming test. *J Pharmacol Exp Ther, 298*, 1269–1279.

Uzunova, V., Sheline, Y., Davis, J. M., Rasmusson, A., Uzunov, D. P., Costa, E., & Guidotti, A. (1998). Increase in the cerebrospinal fluid content of neurosteroids in patients with unipolar major depression who are receiving fluoxetine or fluvoxamine. *Proc Natl Acad Sci USA, 95*, 3239–3244.

van Broekhoven, F., & Verkes, R. J. (2003). Neurosteoids in depression: a review. *Psychopharmacology, 165*, 97-110.

Viau V. (2002). Functional cross-talk between the hypothalamic-pituitary-gonadal and -adrenal axes. *J Neuroendocrinol. 14(6)*, 506-13

Walf, A. A., Rhodes, M. E., & Frye, C. A. (2004). Antidepressant effects of ERbeta-selective estrogen receptor modulators in the forced swim test. *Pharmacol Biochem Behav, 78*, 523-529.

Walker, C. D., Deschamps, S., Proulx, K., Tu, M., Salzman, C., Woodside, B., Lupien, S., Gallo-Payet, N., Richard, D. (2004). Mother to infant or infant to mother? Reciprocal regulation of responsiveness to stress in rodents and the implications for humans. *J Psychiatry Neurosci., 29(5)*, 364-82.

Westenbroek, C., DenBoer, J. A., Veenhuis, M., & TerHorst, G. J. (2004). Chronic stress and social housing differentially affect neurogenesis in male and female rats. *Brain Res. Bull., 64*, 303-308.

Wolkowitz, O. M., Epel, E. S., & Reus V. I. (2001). Stress hormone-related psychopathology: pathophysiological and treatment implications. *World J Biol Psychiatry, 2(3)*, 115-43.

Zonana, J., & Gorman, J. M. (2005). The neurobiology of postpartum depression. *CNS Spectrums, 10(10)*, 792-799.

In: New Research on Postpartum Depression
Editor: Adrian I. Rosenfield, pp. 151-166
ISBN 1-60021-284-0
© 2007 Nova Science Publishers, Inc.

Chapter X

UTILITY OF THE POSTPARTUM DEPRESSION SCREENING SCALE AMONG LOW-INCOME ETHNIC MINORITY WOMEN

Rhonda C. Boyd[*]

University of Pennsylvania School of Medicine and Children's Hospital of Philadelphia

Heidi Worley

Population Reference Bureau, Formerly of Maternity Care Coalition

ABSTRACT

Postpartum depression (PPD) is a serious and common mental health problem. Mothers in low-income families have increased rates of depression, but there is limited information available about PPD in ethnic minority groups. The purpose of this pilot investigation was to assess the psychometric properties and appropriateness of the Postpartum Depression Screening Scale (PDSS) in a community sample of low-income, ethnic minority postpartum women. Seventy-six women (89% ethnic minority) were recruited through a community agency and screened in their homes or community centers. The results showed that the PDSS total score had excellent internal consistency and good construct validity. Fifty-six percent of the women scored above the clinical cut-off score on the PDSS. The PDSS demonstrated some utility limitations, however, as issues of literacy, multiple stressors, and large numbers of women scoring above the clinical cut-off were concerns that arose as potential screening problems for postpartum depression within this population.

Keywords: postpartum depression; screening; ethnic minority

---

[*] Correspondence concerning this chapter should be sent to: Dr. Rhonda Boyd, Department of Psychiatry, Children's Hospital of Philadelphia, 3535 Market Street, Suite 1230, Philadelphia, PA 19104, fax: 215-590-7410, e-mail: rboyd@mail.med.upenn.edu.

INTRODUCTION

Postpartum depression (PPD) is a serious psychiatric disorder that can have negative effects on women, children, and families. PPD has received recent widespread attention in the media as a result of high profile cases and public figures acknowledging that they suffered from the disorder. Additionally, there have been several federal initiatives to increase screening efforts and treatment of PPD (Boyd, Pearson, & Blehar, 2002). In spite of the negative consequences of, frequency of, and increased focus on PPD, there are still huge gaps in our empirical knowledge in this area. This chapter presents a pilot study on the utility of the Postpartum Depression Screening Scale (PDSS) within a low-income, mostly ethnic minority sample of new mothers to address culturally appropriate screening of PDD.

Postpartum Mood Disturbance

Three mood disturbances are frequently noted after childbirth: (1) postpartum blues; (2) postpartum depression (PPD); and (3) postpartum psychosis. Estimates of up to 85% of postpartum women will experience postpartum blues, and there is a period of heightened reactivity that may last up to two weeks after delivery (O'Hara, 1987). PPD has been classified by the Diagnostic Statistical Manual-IV (American Psychiatric Association, 1994) as a subtype of Major Depressive Disorder (MDD) that occurs within 4 weeks after childbirth. MDD is characterized by depressed mood or loss of interest and pleasure for two weeks accompanied by at least four other symptoms including feelings of worthlessness or guilt, appetite changes with weight loss or gain, fatigue, insomnia or over sleeping, difficulty concentrating, suicidal ideation, and feelings of psychomotor agitation or slowness. Approximately 10-15% of women experience PPD (O'Hara, Zekoski, Phillips, & Wright, 1990). Postpartum psychosis is the least common (.001-.002%) and most virulent postpartum mood disorder. It is characterized by delusions, hallucinations, restlessness, irritability, sleep disturbance and mood lability (O'Hara, 1987). Postpartum psychosis often has an abrupt onset when it occurs, and 60% - 79% of women develop it within two weeks following delivery (Chaudron & Pies, 2003)

Of all other chronic diseases, depression places the second greatest burden on women's health worldwide (World Health Organization, 2002). Women who have experienced PPD are at increased risk for future depressive episodes (Cooper & Murray, 1995; Philipps & O'Hara, 1991). Of particular concern is the negative impact PPD can have on the mother-infant relationship and infant development. Depression has been related to poor mother-infant interaction and attachment difficulties (Field, 1998; Martins & Gaffan, 2000). Furthermore, there is considerable evidence of the deleterious effects of maternal depression on an infant's functioning including the domains of cognition, social functioning, and developmental milestones (Goodman & Gotlib, 1999).

Postpartum Depression and Low-Income Women

The extent to which socioeconomic factors influence the risk of PPD is not yet fully appreciated. Rates of PPD for women living in poverty are generally higher than the average, ranging up to 38% (Hobfoll, Ritter, Lavin, Hulsizer, & Cameron, 1995). Some studies have shown rates as high as 50% (McKee, Cunningham, Jankowksi, & Zayas, 2001; Orr & Miller, 1995). Prevalence of prenatal depression, which has been consistently linked to the risk of PPD, is also higher in low-income populations, ranging from 25% to 47% (Bennett, Einarson, Taddio, Keren, & Einarson, 2004).

Postpartum Depression and Ethnic Minority Women

There is limited information available about postpartum depression symptomatology with ethnic minority women. Understanding the expression of depressive symptoms and postpartum experiences, which may vary across cultural groups, is critical for screening and detection (Bashiri & Spielvogel, 1999). An international study (Affonso, De, Horowitz, & Mayberry, 2000) of postpartum women showed great variability among the level of depressive symptoms between and within countries. Specifically, postpartum women from Australia and Europe had the lowest mean scores while women from Asia and South America had the highest. In one study of low-income postpartum women in the U.S., African American women reported higher rates of clinically significant depressive symptoms than Hispanic women at three weeks postpartum, but not at later weeks. Similarly, this study also found that Hispanic women who spoke both English and Spanish were at greatest risk for depressive symptoms than Spanish-only speakers at three weeks postpartum (Yonkers et al., 2001). One study showed that low-income, urban Latina mothers' continued depression from pregnancy to the postpartum period was significantly related to the mother's significant negative life events (Zayas, Jankowski, & McKee, 2003). In a recent qualitative study of African American mothers who experienced PPD, Amankwaa (2003) identified perceived stress, level of family and social support, perception of being overwhelmed, and thoughts of negative dreams, harm and suicide as additional questions to incorporate in screening questionnaires of PPD.

Screening for PPD

The implementation of widespread screening for depression in postpartum women has been recommended (Heneghan, Silver, Bauman, & Stein, 2000; Horowitz, Damato, Solon, von Metzsch, & Gill, 1995). Screening has many benefits including identifying those in need for mental health services and detection of an underserved population. In addition, screening can be a crucial step in the prevention of mental health problems for mothers and their infants (Boyd et al., 2002; Muñoz, Le, & Ghosh Ippen, 2000). Therefore, valid and reliable screening measures are needed.

Few self-report measures exist that specifically assess for postpartum depression symptoms and can be used as screening tools (Boyd, Le, & Somberg, 2005). The most commonly used postpartum depression self-report instrument, the Edinburgh Postpartum Depression Scale (EPDS; Cox, Holden, & Sagovsky, 1987), has extensive and moderate psychometric data available across a diverse array of countries, such as Nigeria, China, and Portugal (e.g., Boyd et al., 2005; Eberhard-Gran, Eskild, Tambs, Opjordsmoen, & Samuelson 2001). Although not as widely used in the U.S., the EPDS has been investigated with inner-city African American and Latina American women (Morris-Rush, Freda, & Bernstein, 2003; Yonkers et al., 2001) and ethnic minority women in England (Onozawa, Kumar, Adams, Dore, & Glover, 2003).

The Postpartum Depression Screening Scale (PDSS; Beck & Gable, 2000) containing 35 items with seven subscales was recently developed to assess symptoms associated with postpartum depression. Psychometric studies conducted by the developers of the PDSS have shown good to high internal consistency (α = .83 to .94) of its subscales (Beck & Gable, 2000). Beck and Gable (2001a) showed the PDSS to be significantly and positively correlated with both the EPDS and the Beck Depression Inventory-II (Beck, Steer, & Brown, 1996), which is a commonly used self-report measure of depression. Comparisons with these other instruments showed that the PDSS had higher sensitivity and specificity for the detection of both major and minor postpartum depression (Beck & Gable, 2001b). However, the PDSS was developed and validated on samples of mostly Caucasian, married, and highly educated women. Recent studies have translated the PDSS into Spanish (Beck, Bernal, & Froman, 2003) and administered the PDSS to screen a mostly Native American, low-income rural sample (Baker et al., 2005). The testing of the PDSS-Spanish version with Latina women demonstrated slightly lower reliability and validity psychometrics than the original PDSS, however, the psychometrics were within an acceptable range (Beck & Gable, 2003; 2005). In the Baker and colleagues (2005) study, findings showed that 23% of their sample scored in the clinically significant range on the PDSS and these women were more likely to have had a history of depression than women who scored in the normative range. There is limited data demonstrating the utility of the PDSS with ethnic minority women. Additional research by other investigators needs to be conducted with diverse samples to further determine the cultural validity of this measure (Boyd et al., 2005)

The purpose of this pilot investigation was to assess the psychometric properties and appropriateness of the PDSS in a community sample of low-income, ethnic minority postpartum women. Specifically, the study examined descriptive information of the PDSS' items, subscales, and total score, assessed the reliability (i.e., internal consistency) of the PDSS' subscales and total score and established construct validity by investigating the relation between the PDSS and other measures of depression.

METHOD

Procedures

The participants were recruited through a community agency that serves women in the areas within and surrounding Philadelphia. A typical client is a low-income pregnant woman or new mother; all women in the area are eligible for services. Participants were eligible if they: 1) were at least 18 years of age; 2) spoke and read English; 3) were between two weeks and three months postpartum; and 4) delivered a live, healthy infant. These criteria correspond with Beck and Gable (2001a; 2001b) criteria for their validation studies of the PDSS. The women were recruited by the staff at a community agency with recruitment flyers describing the study.

The screenings were conducted in conjunction with the community agency services. The research staff either administered the measures at home visits with the agency staff or at one of the agency sites. During the assessments, consent was gathered and the participants completed three depression measures and a demographic form. The participants received a gift certificate to a local department store worth $20 for participation and bus tokens if they used public transportation. The study was approved by the Internal Review Board of the Children's Hospital of Philadelphia.

If a woman endorsed suicidal items on any of the measures during the assessment, follow-up questions were asked to determine her suicidal intent and plan. Although suicidal ideation occurred during the study, no participant was at risk for immediate psychiatric hospitalization. If a participant scored above the cut-off for any of the measures, the first author contacted her agency staff member to inform her of the results so that the staff member could ascertain whether the client wanted treatment. All participants received a list of local mental health services at the screening. On several occasions, the primary author talked with the participant to discuss the results and potential treatment.

Sample Characteristics

One hundred and fourteen women indicated that they were interested in participating in this study by signing a recruitment flyer or verbal consent to the agency staff, but only 80 women were screened (70% participant rate). Of the 34 women who did not participate: 10 were not able to be contacted; nine were not eligible (i.e., could not be scheduled prior to three months postpartum, under 18 years of age); six were no longer interested; five were missed because the project ended; three missed appointments and could not be rescheduled; and one was no longer receiving services from the referring agency.

Seventy-six eligible women completed the assessment. Four additional women completed the screening, but afterwards it was discovered that they did not meet all the eligibility criteria: two women lacked English literacy skills they need to adequately complete the questionnaires; one woman had an infant who was very ill at birth, and one woman was beyond three months postpartum.

Of the 76 women who participated in the study, their ages ranged from 19 to 37 with a mean of 24.89 years (SD= 4.76). The majority of the women were ethnic minority (89.4%, n = 68). The racial/ethnic composition was as follows: 78.9% (n = 60) African American, 10.5% (n = 8) White, 7.9% (n = 6) Latina and 2.6% biracial (one woman was African American and Native American and one woman was White and Native American). Sixty five percent (n = 49) reported being single, 31% (n = 23) were married or living with a partner, 3% (n = 2) were separated or divorced and the remaining 2% (n = 2) identified as other. Forty four percent completed high school or a GED (n = 33), 30% (n = 23) did not complete high school, 21% (n = 16) had vocational training or some college, and 5% (n = 4) completed college. All participants were on public assistance.

The postpartum period ranged from 2.3 weeks to 13.4 weeks with a mean of 6.2 weeks. Eighty-one percent had a vaginal birth. Their number of pregnancies ranged from 1 to 10 with a mean of 3.5 and their number of living children also ranged from 1 to 10 with a mean of 2.6. In regards to breastfeeding, 22% (n = 17) were currently breastfeeding only, 9% (n = 7) were sometimes breastfeeding and 69% (n = 52) were not breastfeeding.

Measures

The Postpartum Depression Screening Scale (PDSS; Beck & Gable, 2000, 2001b, 2002) is a 35-item measure that assesses a total score and seven dimensions of PPD focusing on the new context of motherhood: Sleeping/Eating Disturbances, Anxiety/Insecurity, Emotional Lability, Mental Confusion, Loss of Self, Guilt/Shame, and Contemplating Harming Oneself. Respondents rate the items on a 5-point Likert scale from Strongly Disagree to Strongly Agree for a time period covering the past two weeks. A cut-off score of 60 represents significant symptoms of depression (mild), while a score of 80 represents a positive screening for PPD (major). The first seven items are the Short Form and yield a Short Total score (Beck & Gable, 2002).

The Edinburgh Postnatal Depression Scale (EPDS; Cox, Holden, & Sagovsky, 1987) measures emotional and cognitive symptoms of PPD over the past seven days. EPDS includes 10 items scored from 0 to 3. There has been some variability in the cut-off scores used to indicate a high level of depressive symptoms. As in other studies, this present study used 12 as a cut-off score (Beck & Gable, 2001b; Yonkers et al., 2001).

The Center for Epidemiological Studies Depression Scale (CES-D; Radloff, 1977) consists of 20 items measuring depressive symptoms. The CES-D was developed as an epidemiological measure of depression for community samples. Respondents are asked to indicate how many days during the past week they experienced various depressive symptoms on a range from 0 to 3. A score of 16 is the cut-off score indicating a high level of depressive symptoms.

RESULTS

PDSS Item Frequencies

Frequencies and percentages (as determined by the number and percentage of participants who endorsed a score of 3 [neither agree or disagree] or greater for each items) for the PDSS are presented in Table 1. The most frequently endorsed items were anxiety over baby, feeling like emotions were on a roller coaster and feeling overwhelmed.

Total and Subscale Scores

Table 2 displays the PDSS total, short total and subscale scores, the EPDS total score and the CES-D total score for the eligible participants. An exploratory analysis was conducted that showed women who breastfed consistently or sometimes did not differ on total depression scores on the PDSS from women who had not breastfed ($t = -0.04$, $p > .05$).

Reliability

Cronbach coefficients were calculated to evaluate the internal consistencies of the PDSS subscales and total score, the EPDS and the CES-D. The internal consistency of the PDSS total sores was .96, and the alpha values for the subscales ranged from .74 to .89 (Table 2). The alpha coefficients were .88 and .92 for the EPDS and CES-D respectively.

Construct Validity

Construct validity of the PDSS was assessed by correlations with the other measures of depression, the EPDS and the CES-D (Table 3). The total score of the PDSS was significant and positively correlated with the total scores on the EPDS ($r = 0.81$, $p < .01$) and the CES-D ($r = 0.82$, $p < .01$). In addition, Table 3 displays correlations of the depression measures with demographic characteristics of the mothers.

Clinical Cut-Off and Agreement across Measures

There were 56% (n = 42) of women who scored in the mild and/or major postpartum depression range for the PDSS. More specifically, 31% (n = 23) of the women scored in the major postpartum depression range while 25% (n = 19) of the women scored in the mild depression range. Women who scored above the clinical cut-off scores for the EPDS and CES-D were 25% (n = 19) and 31% (n = 23) respectively.

Table 1. Item Frequencies of the Postpartum Depression Screening Scale

Item	n	%
Anxiety over baby. (ANX)	42	56.8
Emotions on a roller coaster. (ELB)	41	54.7
Feeling overwhelmed. (ANX)	41	54.6
Irritability. (ELB)	36	48.0
Trouble sleeping. (SLP)	35	46.7
Loss of Appetite. (SLP)	35	46.6
Waking up in the middle of the night. (SLP)	33	44.0
Could not eat. (SLP)	31	41.4
Toss and turn while trying to sleep. (SLP)	29	38.7
Feeling alone. (ANX)	27	36.0
Crying for no reason. (ELB)	24	32.1
Feeling like losing mind. (MNT)	22	29.3
Feeling like moving and pacing. (ANX)	22	29.3
Could not concentrate. (MNT)	21	28.1
Not the mother want to be. (GLT)	20	26.7
Thought was going crazy. (MNT)	20	26.7
Scared never be happy again. (ELB)	19	25.3
Difficulty making decision. (MNT)	19	25.3
Afraid that would not be normal self again. (LOS)	18	24.0
Difficulty focusing on task. (MNT)	18	24.0
Feeling like a stranger to self. (LOS)	15	20.0
Feeling like jumping out of skin. (ANX)	15	20.0
Feeling like many mothers better than me. (GLT)	13	17.3
Not know who I was. (LOS)	12	16.0
Feeling anger ready to explode. (ELB)	12	15.9
Not feeling normal. (LOS)	11	14.6
Failure as a mother. (GLT)	11	14.6
Hiding thoughts and feelings toward baby. (GLT)	9	12.0
Not feeling real. (LOS)	8	10.6
Wanting to leave the world. (SUI)	7	9.3
Thinking would be better off dead. (SUI)	5	6.7
Death is the way of out this nightmare. (SUI)	5	6.6
Feeling guilty because could not feel love for baby. (GLT)	5	6.6
Want to hurt myself. (SUI)	4	5.4
Feeling baby would be better off without me. (SUI)	3	4.0

Note: SLP = Sleeping/Eating Disturbances; ANX = Anxiety/Insecurity; ELB = Emotional Lability; MNT = Mental Confusion; LOS = Loss of Self; GLT = Guilt/Shame; SUI = Suicidal Thoughts

PDSS content copyright © 2002 by Western Psychological Services. Items summarized and reprinted by permission of the publisher, Western Psychological Services, 12031 Wilshire Boulevard, Los Angeles, California, 90025, U.S.A. (www.wpspublish.com). Not to be reprinted in whole or in part for any additional purpose without the expressed, written permission of the publisher. All rights reserved.

Table 2. Descriptive Statistics of the Depression Measures

	Mean	SD	Range	α
PDSS				
Total	68.92	27.33	35 - 148	.96
Short Total	15.96	6.47	6 - 33	.83
Sleeping/Eating	12.56	5.65	5 - 25	.85
Anxiety/Insecurity	11.87	4.72	4 - 24	.74
Emotional Lability	11.36	5.07	5 - 23	.85
Mental Confusion	9.85	5.03	5 - 23	.89
Loss of Self	8.84	4.45	5 - 22	.89
Guilt/Shame	8.08	3.94	5 - 20	.83
Suicidal Thoughts	6.39	2.69	5 - 16	.89
Inconsistency Score	1.55	1.41	0 - 5	-
EPDS	7.61	5.89	0 - 22	.88
CES-D	13.87	12.40	0 - 51	.92

Note: CES-D = Center for Epidemiological Studies Depression Scale; EPDS = Edinburgh Postnatal Depression Scale; PDSS = Postpartum Depression Screening Scale

Table 3. Correlations

	1	2	3	4	5	6	7	8
1. PDSS Total								
2. PDSS Short	.91**							
3. EPDS	.81**	.72**						
4. CES-D	.83**	.73**	.83**					
5. Postpartum Weeks	.27*	.24*	.21	.29*				
6. Age of Mother	.19	.18	.16	.11	-.11			
7. Pregnancies (#)	.18	.13	.15	.19	-.07	.51**		
8. Children (#)	.06	-.05	.04	.06	-.02	.56**	.74**	

Note: CES-D = Center for Epidemiological Studies Depression Scale; EPDS = Edinburgh Postnatal Depression Scale; PDSS = Postpartum Depression Screening Scale; # = number; * $p < .05$; ** $p < .01$

There were 30 (39% of the eligible participants) women who scored above the cut-off on at least one of the measures (using the major postpartum depression cut-off for the PDSS). Agreement of the PDSS with the other depression measures varied slightly. Of the thirty women who scored above the clinical level: sixteen women (53.3%) scored high on all measures; four (13.3%) scored high on only the PDSS; and three (10%) scored high on both the PDSS and the CES-D. Seven women (23.3%) were high on either the CES-D or the EPDS. Expanding to include mild depression on the PDSS (n = 19), only three (11%) of the women who scored in the mild range also scored above the clinical cut-off on the other depression instruments. Of the 30 who scored high on any of the measures, seven (23%) indicated that they were interested in treatment or sought treatment after the screening.

Conclusion

The psychometric properties of the PDSS were shown to be adequate in this low income, ethnic minority sample. The internal consistency of the PDSS total score was excellent. Its short scale and subscales demonstrated good internal consistencies, with the exception of the Anxiety/Insecurity subscale that had a moderate coefficient alpha. The PDSS demonstrated construct validity in that it was positively correlated with a measure of postpartum depression and a general measure of depression.

What was most striking in this study is the high number of women who scored in the mild and major depression range on the PDSS. With 56% of the women in this sample scoring in the mild or major depression range, this rate is higher than rates reported in other studies of the PDSS. Namely, 31% of the women scored in the clinical range in a white highly educated sample (Beck & Gable, 2001a), 23.2% in a mostly ethnic minority rural population (Baker et al., 2005), and 37% in a Latina population (Beck & Gable, 2005). Recent review of PDSS screening instruments suggested that the PDSS may be better able to identify women with MDD (Boyd et al., 2005; Gaynes et al., 2005). The rate of women who scored in the major postpartum depression range on the PDSS was similar to the rates of women who scored in the clinical range on the EPDS and CES-D. In another study, the use of the Major Depression cut-off score on the PDSS and 12/13 cut-off score on the EPDS identified the same eight women in an Australian sample (Hanna, Jarman & Savage, 2004). Nevertheless, the rates for this pilot study ranged from 25-31% and are above the estimated prevalence rates for PDD. However, they were consistent with studies finding higher rates of PPD with low-income women (e.g., Hobfoll et al., 1995; Morris-Rush et al., 2003).

Since the majority of the sample was ethnic minority (mostly African American), the implications of this study for race and ethnicity must be considered. This study suggested that more than half of low-income minority postpartum women are exhibiting high levels of depressive symptoms. It has been documented that many U.S. ethnic minority women are commonly exposed to a host of environmental factors that are likely increase their vulnerability to depression, such as poverty, residence in inner-city environments, exposure to violence, and racism (Brown, Abe-Kim, & Carrio, 2003; U.S. Department of Health and Human Services, 2001). In this pilot study, it was difficult to tease out the influence of ethnic minority status from poverty. In one longitudinal study of African American postpartum mothers that spanned socioeconomic statuses, Beeghly and colleagues (2003) found that low-income was related to higher levels of depressive symptoms between 2-18 months after childbirth, suggesting further evidence for the relation between poverty and postpartum depression.

A related issue in this sample is that 30% of the women did not finish high school, with implications for their low-income status, as well their ability to understand the self-report instruments. A range of literacy challenges emerged during the screenings. A handful of clients who were recent immigrants from Caribbean and African countries had trouble understanding some of the items even though they spoke and read English, but it was not their first language. Additionally, native English speakers needed clarification on a number of items across all three instruments and the socioeconomic survey. Although the PDSS was developed for a seventh grade reading level, the most common difficulty was in the participants' understanding of the response set on its Likert scale (e.g., the difference between "strongly agree" and "strongly disagree"). Such literacy problems raise concerns about the content validity of the items and the accuracy of the responses among a low-income population who may have major literacy deficits. In addition, it suggests that having women complete questionnaires by themselves may not be the optimal way to screen for PPD in some populations.

PPD is confounded with life stressors, which this sample reported often during the screenings or follow-up discussions; particularly those whom scored in a clinical range on the self-report instruments. The women expressed multiple life stressors, including those related to: housing/homelessness, financial/work-related, childcare, marital, child health, own health, generalized stressful life events, and generalized feelings of being overwhelmed, which was one of the most frequent items endorsed on the PDSS. Such a high prevalence of life stressors might help explain the unanticipated high proportion of women who scored above the cut-off on any measure. Perhaps the questionnaires are picking up more generalized life stressors that may or may not contribute to clinical PPD. Amankwaa (2003) found that experiencing stressors emerged as a theme and preceded postpartum depression symptoms among African American women. A meta-analytical review also identified stressful life events as a risk factor for PPD (O'Hara & Swain, 1996). The influence of generalized life stressors on PPD needs to be explored through additional research with these instruments in order to fully understand the implications for screening.

Few women scored above the clinical cut-off score sought treatment when recommended. This finding has implications for addressing PPD in the broader population. In this study, only 23% of those for whom treatment was recommended followed through. For some, childcare issues posed a feasibility problem. Mental health treatment programs for low-income mothers need to integrate childcare services into their environments to address this treatment barrier.

There were several limitations to this study. As a pilot study, this investigation was limited in sample size and scope. The sample size was not large enough to conduct confirmatory factor analyses of the PDSS in this population. Structured interviews to confirm the diagnoses of MDD or another depressive disorder were not conducted and thus sensitivity, specificity, positive predictive value and negative predictive values of the PDSS were not calculated. Because the eligibility criteria required that the participants speak and read English, Latina women were less likely to be able to participate in the study. The sample that participated in the study could have exhibited more depressive symptoms than the typical client of the community agency. It is very possible that by informing the community agency staff about the nature of the study, they referred women about whom they had concerns regarding depressive symptoms to the study. They used the study as a resource and service for some of their clients. Additionally, one site recruited more than half of the participants and thus there may be a selection bias. Finally, information regarding the women's history of or treatment for depression was not gathered.

This study lends support for the general utility of the PDSS in screening for depressive symptoms in low-income minority women. However, identified difficulties included the Likert scaling that may not be understood by women with limited literacy and the potentially high number of women who scored in mild and major depression range. With approximately half of low-income ethnic minority women scoring high on the PDSS, considerable effort and follow-up resources may be used for women who may not need it. Only 23% of the women who scored above the cut-off on the screening measures had an interest in or pursued treatment. The use of the Major Depression criteria for postpartum depression cut-off seems to be most appropriate in this population. This pilot study also raises general concerns about PPD screening in this population with potential literacy difficulties and high levels of chronic stressors. Further research is needed to understand how screening instruments work in different populations, as Gaynes and colleagues (2003) also concluded. As the field awaits this research, it is important to use self-report measures of PPD in a way that is congruent and appropriate with the sample.

ACKNOWLEDGEMENTS

This research was supported by grants from the Center of Excellence for Diversity and Health Education and Research at the University of Pennsylvania and the National Institute of Mental Health (K01 MH 068619). The authors thank Maternity Care Coalition for their research collaboration, Jane Pearson for her helpful review and Jameika Sampson, Sarah Hatton Lewis, Gary Colin Emerle, and Jamille Williams for their research assistance.

REFERENCES

Affonso, D. D., De, A. K., Horowitz, J. A., & Mayberry, L. J. (2000). An international study exploring levels of postpartum depressive symptomatology. *Journal of Psychosomatic Research, 29,* 207-216.

Amankwaa, L.C. (2003). Postpartum depression among African-American women. *Issues in Mental Health Nursing, 24,* 297-316.

American Psychiatric Association. (1994). *Diagnostic and statistical manual of mental disorders* (4th ed.). Washington DC: APA.

Baker, L., Cross, S., Greaver, L., Wei, G., Lewis, R., & Healthy Start Corps. (2005). Prevalence of postpartum depression in a Native American population. *Maternal and Child Health Journal, 9,* 21-25.

Bashiri, N., & Spielvogel, A. M. (1999). Postpartum depression: a cross-cultural perspective. *Primary Care Update for the Obstetrician-Gynecologist, 6,* 82-87.

Beck, C. T., Bernal, H., & Froman, R. D. (2003). Methods to document semantic equivalence of a translated scale. *Research in Nursing and Health, 26,* 64-73.

Beck, C. T., & Gable, R. K. (2000). Postpartum Depression Screening Scale: Development and psychometric testing. *Nurse Researcher, 49,* 272-282.

Beck, C. T., & Gable, R. K. (2001a). Further validation of the Postpartum Depression Screening Scale. *Nursing Research, 50,* 155-164.

Beck, C. T., & Gable, R. K. (2001b). Comparative analysis of the performance of the Postpartum Depression Screening Scale with two other depression instruments. *Nursing Research, 50,* 242-250.

Beck, C.T., & Gable, R.K. (2002). Manual for Postpartum Depression Screening Scale. Los Angeles, CA: Western Psychological Services.

Beck, C.T., & Gable, R.K. (2003). Postpartum Depression Screening Scale-Spanish version. *Nursing Research, 52,* 296-306.

Beck, C.T., & Gable, R.K. (2005). Screening performance of the Postpartum Depression Screening Scale-Spanish version. *Journal of Transcultural Nursing, 16,* 331-338.

Beck, A. T., Steer, R. A., & Brown, G. K. (1996). *Manual for Beck Depression Inventory-II.* San Antonio Texas: Psychological Corporation.

Beeghly, M., Olson, K. L., Weinberg, M. K., Pierre, S.C., Downey, N., & Tronick, E.Z. (2003). Prevalence, stability, and socio-demographic correlates of depressive symptoms in black mothers during the first 18 months postpartum. *Maternal & Child Health Journal, 7,* 157-168.

Bennett, H. A., Einarson, A., Taddio, A., Keren, G., & Einarson, T. R. (2004). Prevalence of depression during pregnancy: systematic review. *Obstetrics and Gynecology, 203,* 698-709.

Boyd, R.C., Le, H.N., & Somberg, R. (2005). Review of screening instruments for postpartum depression. *Archives of Women's Mental Health, 8,* 141-153.

Boyd, R.C., Pearson, J.L., & Blehar, M.C. (2002). Prevention and treatment of depression in pregnancy and the postpartum period-summary of a maternal depression roundtable: A U.S. perspective. *Archives of Women's Mental Health, 4,* 79-83.

Brown, C., Abe-Kim, J. S., & Carrio, C. (2003). Depression in ethnically diverse women: implications for treatment in primary care settings. *Professional Psychology: Research and Practice, 34,* 10-19.

Chaudron, L. H., & Pies RW. (2003). The relationship between postpartum psychosis and bipolar disorder: a review. *Journal of Clinical Psychiatry, 64,* 1284-1292.

Cooper, P. J., & Murray, L. (1995). Course and recurrence of postnatal depression: evidence for the specificity of the diagnostic concept. *British Journal of Psychiatry, 166,* 191-195.

Cox J. L., Holden, J.M., & Sagovsky, R. (1987). Detection of postnatal depression: Development of the 10-item Edinburgh Postnatal Depression Scale. *The British Journal of Psychiatry: the Journal of Mental Science, 150,* 782-786.

Eberhard-Gran, M., Eskild, A., Tambs, K., Opjordsmoen, S., & Samuelson, S. O. (2001). Review of the validation studies of the Edinburgh Postnatal Depression Scale. *Acta Psychiatrica Scandinavica, 104,* 243-249.

Field, T. (1998). Maternal depression effects on infants and early interventions. *Preventive Medicine, 27,* 200-203.

Gaynes, B. N., Gavin, N., Meltzer-Brody, S., Lohr, K. N., Swinson, T., Gartlehner, G., Brody, S., Miller, W. C. (2005). Perinatal depression: Prevalence, screening accuracy, and screening outcomes. *Summary, Evidence Report/Technology Assessment No. 119.*

AHRQ Publication No. 05-E006-1. Rockville, MD: Agencry for Healthcare Research and Quality.

Goodman, S.H., & Gotlib, I.H. (1999). Risk for psychopathology in children of depressed mothers: a developmental model for understanding mechanisms of transmission. *Psychological Review, 106,* 458-490.

Hanna, B., Jarman, H., & Savage, S. (2004). The clinical application of three screening tools for recognizing post-partum depression. *International Journal of Nursing Practice, 10,* 72-79.

Heneghan, A. M., Silver, E. J., Bauman, L. J., & Stein, R. E. K. (2000) Do pediatricians recognize mothers with depressive symptoms? *Pediatrics, 106,* 1367-1373.

Hobfoll, S. E., Ritter, C., Lavin, J., Hulsizer, M. R., & Cameron, R. P. (1995). Depression prevalence and incidence among inner-city pregnant and postpartum women. *Journal of Consulting and Clinical Psychology, 63,* 445-53.

Horowitz, J. A., & Damato, E., Solon, L., von Metzsch, G., & Gill, V. (1995). Postpartum depression: Issues in clinical assessment. *Journal of Perinatology, 16,* 268-278.

Martins, C., & Gaffan, E. A. (2000). Effects of early maternal depression on patterns of infant-mother attachment: a meta-analytic investigation. *Journal of Child Psychology and Psychiatry, 41,* 737-746.

McKee, M. D., Cunningham, D., Jankowksi, K. R. B., & Zayas, L. H. (2001). Health-related functional status in pregnancy: relationship to depression and social support in a multi-ethnic population. *Obstetrics and Gynecology, 97,* 988-93.

Morris-Rush, J. K, Freda, M.C., & Bernstein, P.S. (2003). Screening for postpartum depression in an inner-city population. *American Journal of Obstetrics and Gynecology, 188,* 1217-1219.

Muñoz, R. F., Le, H. N, & Ghosh Ippen, C. (2000). We should screen for major depression. *Applied and Preventive Psychology, 9,* 123-133.

O'Hara, M. W. (1987). Post-partum blues, depression and psychosis: A review. *Journal of Psychosomatic Obstetrics Gynecology, 7,* 205-227.

O'Hara, M. W., Zekoski, E. M., Phillips, L. H., & Wright, E. J. (1990). A controlled prospective study of postpartum mood disorders: Comparisons of childbearing and nonchildbearing women. *Journal of Abnormal Psychology, 99,* 3-15.

O'Hara, M. W., & Swain, A. M., 1996. Rates and risk of postpartum depression-A meta-analysis. *International Review of Psychiatry, 8,* 37-54.

Onozawa, K., Kumar, R.C., Adams, D., Dore, C., & Glover, V. (2003). High EPDS scores in women from ethnic minorities living in London. *Archives of Women's Mental Health, 6(Suppl 2),* 51-55.

Orr, S. T., & Miller, C. A. (1995). Maternal depressive symptoms and the risk of poor pregnancy outcome: review of the literature and preliminary findings. *Epidemiologic Reviews, 17,* 165-71.

Philipps, L. H., & O'Hara, M. W. (1991). Prospective study of postpartum depression: 4 1/2-year follow-up of women and children. *Journal of Abnormal Psychology, 100,* 151-155.

Radloff, L. S. (1977). The CES-D Scale: A self-report depression scale for research in the general population. *Applied Psychological Measurement, 1,* 385-401.

U.S. Department of Health and Human Services (2001). *Mental health: Culture, Race, and Ethnicity-A supplement to mental health: A report of the Surgeon General.* Rockville, MD: U.S. Department of Health and Human Services, Substance Abuse and Mental Health Services Administration, Center for Mental Health Services.

World Health Organization (2002). *The World Health Report 2002: reducing risks, promoting healthy life.* World Health Organization, Geneva, Switzerland.

Yonkers, K. A., Ramin, S. M., Rush, A. J., Navarrete, C. A., Carmody, T., March, D., Hearwell, SF., & Leveno, K.J. (2001). Onset and persistence of postpartum depression in an inner-city maternal health clinic system. *The American Journal of Psychiatry, 158,* 1856-1863.

Zayas, L. H., Jankowski, K. R. B. (2003). Prenatal and postpartum depression among low-income Dominican and Puerto Rican women. *Hispanic Journal of Behavioral Sciences, 25,* 370-385.

INDEX

A

acceptance, 14, 17, 18, 20, 42
access, 40, 42, 50, 54
acculturation, viii, 24, 30, 42, 45
accuracy, 55, 99, 161, 163
ACTH, 6, 77, 79, 134
activity level, 139
adaptation, viii, x, 7, 12, 24, 29, 33, 105, 117, 118
adjustment, vii, 1, 2, 4, 5, 9, 10, 11, 13, 15, 16, 17, 18, 19, 115, 119, 127
adolescence, x, 105, 108
adult population, 54
adulthood, xi, 10, 131, 133
adults, 15, 119
aetiology, 122, 123
affect, xi, 10, 16, 17, 48, 61, 62, 72, 73, 75, 102, 127, 132, 149
affective disorder, ix, 2, 31, 70, 72, 73, 75, 77, 78, 79, 83, 91, 93, 148
African American women, 153, 161
age, 3, 10, 37, 39, 40, 42, 48, 61, 70, 91, 102, 108, 110, 111, 112, 114, 115, 124, 133, 140, 148, 155
aggression, 5, 23, 24, 26, 139
alternative, 129
alters, 147, 148
American Psychiatric Association, 152, 162
American Psychological Association, 27
androgens, 21
anemia, 35, 98
anger, 158
animals, 6, 7, 9, 135, 136, 141
ANS, 144

antidepressant, ix, 59, 90, 91, 96, 97, 98, 99, 103, 135, 141, 146, 147, 148, 149
anxiety, xi, 3, 9, 16, 33, 35, 48, 49, 51, 53, 54, 55, 56, 57, 63, 73, 74, 83, 98, 118, 119, 122, 127, 129, 131, 136, 139, 141, 145, 157
anxiety disorder, xi, 122, 131
appetite, 152
appraisals, 108
Argentina, 43
argument, 4, 16, 122, 123
arousal, 7
Asia, 153
assessment, viii, 3, 29, 30, 31, 32, 33, 35, 43, 51, 55, 56, 91, 99, 124, 155
association, x, 12, 30, 37, 38, 39, 40, 41, 78, 105, 106, 110, 114, 115, 126, 135, 138
attachment, vii, 1, 2, 6, 7, 9, 10, 17, 19, 21, 27, 28, 87, 101, 102, 115, 118, 120, 147, 152, 164
attention, 35, 52, 60, 65, 98, 107, 152
attitudes, 119
attractiveness, 138
attribution, 17
Australia, 49, 54, 64, 66, 121, 123, 129, 153
availability, viii, 16, 29
awareness, 123

B

barriers, ix, 59, 60, 61, 63, 64, 65
Beck Depression Inventory, 32, 37, 41, 154, 163
behavior, 5, 7, 9, 10, 11, 19, 20, 21, 22, 23, 24, 25, 26, 27, 35, 102, 118, 119, 134, 136, 139, 140, 142, 143, 144, 145, 147, 148
behavioral models, 25

benign, x, 30, 33, 86, 97
bias, 8, 11, 14, 99, 127, 161
binding, 20, 24
binding globulin, 20
bipolar disorder, 74, 79, 82, 88, 163
birth, vii, ix, xi, 1, 2, 3, 5, 6, 7, 10, 14, 15, 16, 17, 18, 32, 36, 37, 38, 40, 43, 59, 87, 92, 101, 107, 116, 117, 121, 122, 139, 140, 155, 156
birth weight, 7
births, viii, 15, 29, 79
blame, 17
blood, 75
blood stream, 75
body, 83, 137
body weight, 83
bonding, 6, 24, 118
bonds, 18
boys, 120
brain, 6, 7, 78, 132, 133, 134, 137, 138, 139, 141, 142, 144, 145, 146, 148
brainstem, 7
Brazil, viii, 29, 30, 31, 34, 38, 39, 42
breakdown, 17
breast milk, 61
breastfeeding, ix, 59, 63, 86, 97, 119, 156

C

California, 37, 118, 158
Canada, 14, 16, 28
candidates, 6
caregivers, 64
caregiving, 12, 13
Caribbean, 31, 160
causality, 116
cell, 136, 137, 140
Census, 30, 46
central nervous system, 21, 134, 140, 141
cerebrospinal fluid, 149
certificate, 155
cervix, 9
child development, v, x, 56, 101, 105, 106, 117, 119
childcare, 16, 134, 161
childhood, x, 10, 17, 23, 42, 105
children, viii, x, xi, 3, 10, 13, 17, 18, 30, 34, 35, 37, 38, 39, 42, 43, 48, 56, 57, 63, 86, 87, 91, 99, 101, 103, 105, 106, 107, 110, 112, 114, 115, 117, 118, 119, 120, 131, 132, 139, 142, 152, 156, 164
Chile, viii, 29, 31, 32, 34, 38, 39, 40, 43, 44, 45
China, 15, 154

cholesterol, 140, 141
circulation, 75
classes, 123, 130
classification, 125
clients, 160, 161
clinical assessment, x, 50, 51, 105, 164
clinical depression, 75
clinical presentation, 2, 101
clinical trials, 86, 138
CNS, 4, 5, 7, 9, 142, 149
cognition, 133, 134, 143, 152
cognitive ability, xi, 131
cognitive development, viii, x, 47, 106, 107, 110, 112, 114, 116, 117, 120
cognitive function, 143
cognitive style, 19
cohort, ix, 54, 57, 73, 85, 86, 87, 88, 91, 93, 94, 97, 98, 100, 103
colic, vii, 1, 18, 40
collaboration, 162
commitment, 5, 10
communication, 52, 67, 137, 140
community, xii, 13, 18, 49, 54, 56, 57, 62, 66, 88, 100, 118, 151, 154, 155, 156, 161
community support, 13
comorbidity, 57
compensation, ix, 59
competence, 5, 8, 9, 11, 18, 41, 42, 52, 120
complement, xi, 122
complexity, 80, 116
complications, 16, 108, 118
components, 80
composition, 156
comprehension, 107
concentration, 60, 76, 77
conception, 108
concordance, 108
conduct, 106, 116, 161
confidence, vii, 2, 11, 13, 19, 126
conflict, 15, 40, 41, 42
confusion, 2, 8, 108, 111
consensus, 49, 63, 102, 109
consent, 155
construct validity, xii, 151, 154, 160
continuity, 18
contraceptives, 9
control, x, 3, 7, 8, 10, 25, 43, 78, 89, 105, 106, 109, 110, 136, 139, 140
control group, x, 10, 43, 89, 105, 106, 109, 110
controlled studies, 86

controlled trials, 49
convergence, 138
coping, v, x, xi, 17, 44, 121, 122, 123, 124, 125, 126, 127, 128, 139
coping strategy, 122
correlation, 16, 41, 108, 111, 112
correlation coefficient, 111, 112
corticotropin, 83, 134, 143, 146
cortisol, ix, xi, 6, 7, 20, 23, 69, 70, 75, 76, 77, 79, 80, 83, 84, 131, 132, 134, 137, 138, 142, 143
Costa Rica, 35, 38, 40
costs, 54, 57
counseling, 61
couples, 15, 34, 36, 123, 124
covering, 156
criticism, 106
crying, 6, 12, 33, 35, 73, 79, 123
cues, 6, 7, 10, 18
cultural norms, 15
cultural practices, vii, 1, 15, 18
culture, 13, 15, 17, 20, 22
cycles, 9, 19

D

database, 31
deficiency, 35, 80, 98, 103, 142
deficit, 133, 137
definition, 99, 103
delivery, vii, x, 3, 4, 7, 8, 9, 10, 15, 16, 18, 19, 35, 39, 42, 54, 61, 78, 79, 88, 93, 97, 99, 105, 126, 133, 152
delusions, 152
demand, 123
demographic characteristics, 22, 37, 91, 157
demographics, 11
density, 137, 140
Department of Defense, 65
Department of Health and Human Services, 67, 160, 165
dependent variable, 108
depressive symptomatology, 3, 10, 12, 14, 16, 17, 19, 21, 22, 26, 34, 43, 89, 101, 143, 162
depressive symptoms, 3, 4, 13, 16, 17, 21, 33, 34, 35, 36, 37, 40, 42, 44, 45, 53, 56, 72, 74, 78, 82, 87, 88, 89, 98, 99, 101, 102, 113, 120, 132, 133, 135, 136, 137, 138, 139, 140, 141, 153, 156, 160, 161, 162, 163, 164
deprivation, 14, 18, 27, 40, 122
desensitization, 28

desire, 14, 61
detection, 32, 49, 51, 52, 54, 56, 62, 99, 153, 154
developed countries, viii, 29, 30
developing countries, 52, 56
developmental milestones, 152
dexamethasone suppression test, 75
Diagnostic and Statistical Manual of Mental Disorders, 88
diagnostic criteria, xi, 34, 89, 90, 106, 113, 122, 127, 128
Diagnostic Statistical Manual, 152
diet, 108, 113
differentiation, 21
direct observation, x, 106, 108, 113
disability, 48
discrimination, 22, 33
disorder, vii, x, xii, 2, 8, 19, 28, 30, 31, 33, 40, 41, 48, 65, 73, 74, 75, 77, 80, 81, 86, 88, 89, 90, 97, 98, 102, 103, 109, 117, 119, 132, 142, 152, 161
disposition, 135
dissatisfaction, 15, 17, 42
distress, 51, 53, 55, 122, 123, 127, 128, 129
diversity, 43, 45, 56
dopamine, 7, 8, 9, 21, 28, 84
dopamine agonist, 8
drug treatment, 82
drugs, 86, 146, 148
DSM, ix, 31, 32, 35, 36, 37, 39, 40, 41, 85, 86, 88, 89, 91, 93, 94, 95, 96, 100, 102, 122
DSM-II, 32, 35, 36, 39
DSM-III, 32, 35, 36, 39
DSM-IV, ix, 31, 32, 35, 37, 40, 41, 85, 86, 88, 89, 91, 93, 94, 95, 96, 100, 102, 122
duration, xi, 2, 3, 20, 48, 53, 55, 86, 89, 90, 94, 95, 99, 101, 109, 110, 111, 112, 113, 114, 115, 116, 119, 121, 123, 124, 125, 128, 133, 136, 148
dysphoria, 3, 33, 38, 40, 41, 84

E

eating, 3
ecology, 18
economic problem, 40
economic status, 38
educated women, 154
educational programs, 64, 65
emission, 102
emotion, 17
emotional disorder, 22, 24, 25, 116
emotional distress, 81

emotional well-being, 11, 86
emotions, 157
employment, 21, 23, 91, 92
employment status, 21, 91, 92
endocrine, 4, 10, 23, 78, 82, 83, 140, 147
endocrine glands, 140
endocrinology, 6
endorphins, 6
energy, vii, 64
England, 21, 26, 31, 66, 154
enrollment, 61
environment, viii, 2, 4, 15, 18, 19, 45, 74
environmental factors, 138, 160
epidemiology, 19, 31, 33
estimating, 3
estrogen, xi, 5, 7, 8, 20, 21, 75, 78, 79, 80, 83, 132, 135, 136, 137, 138, 147, 148
ethnic minority, xii, 151, 152, 153, 154, 156, 160, 162
ethnicity, 37, 40, 42, 160
etiology, ix, xi, 2, 11, 69, 78, 81, 132, 134, 139, 140, 141, 142, 143
Europe, 14, 16, 153
evidence, viii, ix, 4, 6, 8, 9, 12, 17, 30, 47, 48, 49, 50, 51, 53, 54, 55, 60, 61, 69, 72, 74, 77, 78, 81, 86, 133, 137, 152, 160, 163
evolution, 5, 28, 97, 100
examinations, 4, 48, 61, 64
exclusion, 107
exercise, 98, 115
expectations, 14, 15, 38, 43
expenditures, 87
expertise, 88
experts, 61, 63
exposure, 6, 7, 9, 42, 50, 61, 97, 138, 160
expression, xi, 4, 6, 16, 26, 114, 131, 136, 147, 153
expulsion, 9, 134

F

failure, 4, 17, 61
failure to thrive, 61
false negative, 3, 53, 56
false positive, 4, 53
family, viii, xi, 4, 13, 14, 15, 18, 29, 37, 38, 39, 40, 41, 42, 43, 47, 51, 52, 61, 62, 75, 79, 82, 87, 93, 98, 108, 118, 121, 123, 126, 127, 128, 132, 153
family history, 75, 82, 93, 98
family income, 39
family members, xi, 18, 121, 126, 127

family physician, 61, 62
family support, 37, 43, 118
fatigue, xi, 3, 60, 121, 152
FDA, 63
fear, ix, 50, 59, 60, 63, 65, 86, 145
feedback, 83
feedback inhibition, 83
feelings, vii, ix, 6, 15, 17, 28, 33, 42, 53, 59, 63, 152, 158, 161
females, 5, 6, 9, 42, 140
fetus, 9, 20
fever, 42
financial resources, viii, 29
floating, 139
flood, 6
fluctuations, xi, 131, 132, 133, 134
fluoxetine, 61, 149
fluvoxamine, 149
focusing, xi, 122, 123, 128, 132, 156, 158
forebrain, 7, 147
forgetting, 42
freedom, 114
friends, 15, 38, 60
funding, 52, 142
funds, 67

G

gender, 22, 38, 39, 87, 98
gender differences, 98
gene, 75, 79, 81, 147
General Health Questionnaire, 3
generation, 78
genetic factors, 12
gestation, ix, 6, 7, 28, 69, 70, 75, 76, 77, 82, 136
gestational age, 6
gift, 155
grants, 162
Great Britain, 2, 14, 19
groups, viii, xii, 24, 30, 128, 137, 151, 153
growth, 8, 9, 24, 61, 66, 79, 83, 137
growth factor, 137
growth hormone, 9, 24, 79, 83
guidelines, x, 51, 55, 86, 100
guilt, vii, 152
guilty, 158

H

hallucinations, 152
happiness, 130
harm, 153
health, viii, 11, 16, 40, 41, 42, 43, 44, 47, 48, 49, 50, 51, 52, 53, 54, 55, 56, 57, 60, 63, 87, 98, 118, 123, 126, 127, 128, 132, 152, 153, 161, 165
health care, viii, 40, 44, 47, 49, 50, 51, 52, 53, 54, 55, 60, 87, 118
health care professionals, 51, 52, 54
health problems, 153
health services, viii, 42, 47, 48, 52, 57, 128
height, 135
heterogeneity, 33
high school, 40, 156, 160
higher education, 89
hippocampus, xi, 132, 133, 137, 143, 145, 146, 148
Hispanic population, 46
Hispanics, 30, 37
homelessness, 161
hopelessness, 15
hormone, vi, ix, xi, 6, 8, 9, 23, 25, 69, 75, 82, 83, 131, 132, 133, 134, 135, 136, 141, 143, 144, 145, 146, 148, 149
hospitalization, 155
hospitals, 35, 36
host, 160
hostility, 106
housing, 161
HPA axis, 8, 75, 76, 132, 133, 134, 138, 141
human brain, 149
human chorionic gonadotropin, 6
husband, 10
hypothalamus, 6, 7, 8, 23, 75, 98, 147
hypothesis, 79, 97, 107, 135
hysterectomy, 27

I

ICD, 34, 36, 39, 41, 90
identification, 3
ideology, 14
idiopathic, 21
imitation, 106
immigrants, 37, 160
immigration, 129
immunoreactivity, 7, 22, 28
implementation, 49, 54, 153
in transition, 57
in vitro, 144
incentives, 65
incidence, 2, 7, 13, 16, 23, 60, 61, 94, 95, 97, 100, 101, 103, 117, 132, 164
inclusion, 3, 96, 98, 107
income, xii, 14, 16, 39, 44, 99, 151, 152, 153, 154, 155, 160, 161, 162, 165
independence, 25
independent variable, 108
India, 15
indirect effect, 10
individual character, 9
induction, 6
industrialized countries, 30
infancy, xi, 10, 108, 131, 132
infant mortality, 8
infants, 4, 5, 6, 9, 10, 12, 13, 14, 16, 18, 21, 23, 27, 35, 52, 61, 63, 64, 81, 102, 117, 119, 120, 134, 138, 144, 153, 163
infection, 39
influence, x, 18, 49, 51, 75, 88, 90, 105, 107, 115, 116, 137, 143, 153, 160, 161
informed consent, 49, 88, 107
injections, 9, 137, 139, 140, 145
insecurity, 87, 102
insight, 2, 142
insomnia, 3, 152
instability, 7
instruction, 15
instrumental support, 14, 16, 17
instruments, viii, 3, 29, 31, 32, 33, 34, 43, 47, 99, 154, 160, 161, 162, 163
insurance, 63
integration, 27
intelligence, 119
intensity, 3, 97
intensive care unit, 102
intent, 155
interaction, x, 6, 10, 11, 26, 31, 51, 101, 106, 108, 109, 112, 113, 114, 116, 117, 119, 120, 128, 141, 152
interactions, 7, 12, 13, 22, 23, 30, 61, 87, 106, 112, 114, 117, 118, 119, 120, 132, 137, 143
interest, ix, 47, 52, 59, 77, 87, 91, 107, 152, 162
interface, 27
interference, 109, 110
internal consistency, xii, 151, 154, 157, 160
International Classification of Diseases, 34, 41
interpersonal relations, 17

interpersonal relationships, 17
interval, 81, 96, 99
intervention, 43, 45, 49, 50, 51, 52, 54, 55, 63, 86, 116, 118, 129, 130
interview, x, 3, 35, 36, 49, 50, 51, 53, 54, 73, 87, 88, 89, 99, 100, 105, 108, 124, 127
intimacy, 10
investment, 27
Iran, 19
iron, 35
irritability, 12, 13, 35, 79, 152
isolation, vii, 1, 2, 14, 18, 122, 123, 138
isotope, 148

J

Jamaica, 15
Japan, 17, 20
Jordan, 13, 23, 123, 129
judgment, 54

K

knowledge, ix, x, 22, 59, 60, 61, 65, 86, 97, 99, 142, 152

L

labor, 5, 7, 8, 9, 15, 16, 18, 20, 23, 25
lack of confidence, xi, 12, 121, 127
lactation, 4, 5, 7, 18, 23, 27, 61, 65, 144
language, viii, 29, 30, 31, 43, 87, 161
language development, 87
latency, 5, 7, 9
Latino women, viii, 30, 31, 42
Latinos, 30
lead, 2, 3, 5, 52, 133, 135, 139
learning, 138, 144
Lebanon, 15, 20
lesions, 6
liability, 60
liberation, 23
LIFE, ix, 85, 88, 89, 90, 98
life cycle, 144
life experiences, 18
life span, 83
lifetime, 39, 93
likelihood, ix, 17, 86, 127
limbic system, 6, 7

limitation, 99, 116, 127
links, 5, 8
listening, 50, 51
literacy, xii, 151, 155, 160, 162
lithium, 90
locus, 78
loneliness, 15
longitudinal study, ix, 10, 11, 85, 101, 118, 160
long-term retention, 19
loss of appetite, 74
love, 158
low risk, 16

M

major depression, x, 8, 24, 35, 48, 51, 62, 83, 86, 87, 99, 100, 101, 102, 103, 132, 133, 137, 141, 143, 146, 147, 148, 149, 160, 162, 164
major depressive disorder, 56, 102, 135
males, 5, 114, 140
management, 54, 87, 97, 98, 100, 107
mania, 74, 80
manic, 73, 79, 80
marital conflict, 38, 48
marital life, 39
marital partners, 17
marital status, 3, 92, 108
marriage, 126
mass, 148
mass spectrometry, 148
mastery, 42
maternal mood, 12, 20, 55, 119, 129
maternal support, 18
meanings, 25
measurement, 2, 3, 10, 28, 45, 73, 82
measures, 78, 83, 153, 154, 155, 156, 157, 159, 162
media, 152
median, x, 86, 94, 95, 97, 98, 100
mediation, 11
medication, 48, 50, 63, 65, 80, 97, 122
memory, 138, 145
men, xi, 34, 98, 101, 121, 122, 123, 124, 125, 126, 127, 128, 132, 135
menarche, 148
menopause, 135, 148
mental disorder, 30, 84, 86, 88, 127, 162
mental health, ix, xii, 41, 42, 47, 48, 49, 50, 51, 52, 55, 56, 57, 63, 83, 118, 127, 151, 153, 155, 165
mental illness, 24, 41, 49, 51, 53, 60, 63, 65, 75, 122
messenger RNA, 26

meta analysis, 57
metabolism, 149
metabolites, 140, 141
Mexico, 18, 42
mice, 23, 27, 133, 137, 143, 144, 145, 146, 148, 149
midbrain, 144
middle class, 15
Middle East, 15
migration, viii, 29, 30
milk, 6, 8
minorities, 50, 164
minority, xii, 151, 160, 162
mobility, 14
models, vi, xi, 19, 78, 131, 132, 133, 134, 135, 140, 141, 142, 146
moderates, 18
modern society, 14
money, 126
mood, vii, viii, ix, xi, 1, 2, 3, 7, 9, 10, 14, 15, 16, 17, 19, 20, 22, 23, 25, 26, 29, 30, 35, 36, 45, 48, 57, 60, 61, 69, 73, 75, 78, 79, 81, 82, 83, 90, 99, 101, 119, 120, 122, 128, 129, 134, 135, 141, 143, 144, 145, 147, 148, 152, 164
mood change, ix, 19, 35, 69, 78, 83, 141, 145
mood disorder, viii, xi, 20, 26, 29, 30, 35, 45, 48, 57, 60, 78, 83, 101, 122, 134, 144, 147, 152, 164
mood states, vii, 1, 2, 10
morbidity, viii, 29, 30, 49, 54, 55, 86
mortality, 49, 86
mothers, v, vii, viii, x, xi, 4, 6, 7, 8, 10, 11, 12, 13, 14, 15, 16, 17, 18, 19, 20, 21, 22, 23, 27, 30, 35, 42, 43, 44, 48, 49, 52, 60, 61, 62, 63, 64, 65, 73, 81, 82, 83, 84, 86, 87, 89, 90, 91, 97, 98, 99, 100, 101, 102, 103, 105, 107, 108, 110, 111, 113, 114, 115, 117, 118, 119, 120, 121, 122, 123, 126, 128, 129, 131, 132, 138, 139, 142, 144, 149, 152, 153, 157, 158, 160, 161, 163, 164
motivation, vii, 1, 2, 4, 5, 7, 10
motor activity, 6
multi-ethnic, 117, 164

N

National Health Service, 54
National Institutes of Health, 67
needs, 6, 12, 13, 16, 38, 43, 51, 52, 53, 63, 123, 154, 161
negative consequences, 152
negativity, 12
neglect, 4

nervous system, 143
network, 41
neurobiology, 149
neurodegeneration, 149
neuroendocrine system, 27
neurogenesis, vi, xi, 131, 132, 133, 134, 136, 139, 140, 143, 145, 146, 147, 148, 149
neuronal cells, 7
neurons, 8, 23
neurophysiology, 10
neurotransmitter, 9, 78
New Zealand, 20, 23, 129
Nigeria, 154
normal development, 8
nucleus, 25, 144
nurses, 43, 50, 52
nursing, 119, 139

O

objectivity, 113
observations, 103, 108
oil, 137, 139, 140
opioids, 18
orchestration, 18
organizations, 64, 65
outpatients, 99
output, 75, 76
ovariectomy, 135, 143, 147
ovulation, 133, 147

P

pacing, 158
pain, 18, 122
panic disorder, 9
paralysis, 9
paranoia, vii
parental care, 8
parental relationships, 17
parental support, 15
parenthood, 20, 48, 51, 101, 124, 129
parenting, 4, 10, 11, 13, 15, 20, 28, 43, 119, 120
parents, x, xi, 15, 16, 18, 19, 43, 47, 52, 121, 123, 126, 127, 128
paroxetine, 63
pathology, 41
pathophysiology, 73, 141, 143
pathways, 50, 51, 54

patient education program, 64
peptides, 6
perceptions, vii, 2, 11, 12, 17, 19, 103, 119, 123
perinatal, viii, ix, 3, 4, 6, 13, 20, 29, 30, 34, 47, 48, 49, 50, 51, 54, 55, 60, 69, 70, 73, 74, 81, 83, 87, 108, 137, 146
permit, 116
personal accounts, 64
personal history, 79
personality, 117, 128
perspective, 20, 24, 28, 48, 51, 54, 83, 98, 99, 127, 129, 130, 162, 163
Peru, viii, 29, 31, 33, 35, 38, 40
pharmacological treatment, 50, 54, 97
pharmacotherapy, 63
physical health, 126
physiology, 148
pilot study, 80, 103, 152, 160, 161, 162
placebo, 8, 83
placenta, 6, 75, 133, 134, 135
planning, 52, 91, 92
plasma, ix, 24, 69, 75, 77, 83, 141, 145, 149
plasma levels, 141
plasticity, 7, 8, 26, 133
pleasure, 152
PM, 66
policy makers, 52
politics, 116
polymorphism, 75, 81
poor, viii, 2, 12, 17, 19, 42, 126, 152, 164
population, xii, 3, 4, 26, 30, 33, 34, 52, 62, 75, 98, 151, 153, 160, 161, 162, 164
Portugal, 154
positive attitudes, 64
positive regard, vii, 1, 19
post traumatic stress disorder, 79
posttraumatic stress, 74, 77, 80, 81
poverty, 14, 153, 160
prediction, 22, 54
predictors, 17, 24, 25, 42, 81, 82, 134, 143
preference, 7, 38
pregnancy, vii, viii, ix, x, xi, 1, 4, 5, 6, 7, 8, 9, 10, 11, 14, 15, 16, 18, 19, 20, 22, 23, 25, 27, 28, 29, 30, 32, 38, 39, 40, 41, 43, 48, 49, 60, 61, 62, 63, 64, 65, 69, 70, 72, 73, 74, 75, 76, 78, 80, 81, 82, 83, 86, 88, 90, 91, 93, 98, 99, 100, 101, 103, 107, 124, 128, 131, 132, 133, 134, 135, 136, 138, 143, 145, 148, 153, 163, 164
prematurity, vii, 1, 18
premenstrual syndrome, 9, 78, 81

preschool, 102, 117
preschool children, 102, 117
prevention, 48, 49, 50, 57, 100, 107, 116, 118, 123, 153
primate, 5
priming, 6, 7, 9
probability, 87, 91, 94, 97, 98
production, 133
progesterone, ix, 5, 8, 9, 18, 21, 69, 75, 78, 79, 80, 132, 133, 134, 135, 136, 137, 138, 140, 141, 143
prognosis, x, 24, 86, 87, 99, 100
program, 37, 43, 53, 54, 64
prolactin, 5, 8, 18
proliferation, 136, 137, 140
prophylactic, 21, 80
prophylaxis, 78
proposition, 10
protective factors, 10
protocol, 88, 90
psychiatric disorders, 13, 20, 35, 55, 86, 89, 101, 116, 132
psychiatric illness, 80, 88, 93
psychiatric morbidity, 19, 84, 101
psychiatrist, 88, 90
psychobiology, 4, 5, 27
psychological distress, 8, 14
psychological health, viii, 2, 19
psychological stress, 11
psychological well-being, 12
psychologist, 88
psychology, 21
psychometric properties, xii, 32, 33, 49, 127, 151, 154, 160
psychopathology, 21, 88, 102, 147, 149, 164
psychoses, 24
psychosis, vii, xi, 5, 8, 10, 14, 24, 27, 28, 30, 34, 48, 57, 73, 74, 75, 78, 79, 80, 81, 82, 84, 131, 152, 163, 164
psychosocial factors, 4, 74
psychosocial functioning, 28, 101
psychosocial stress, vii, 1, 8, 17, 18
psychosocial support, 14, 15
psychotherapy, 50, 99
psychotic symptoms, 88, 98
public awareness, 64
public health, 48
public sector, 54

Q

qualitative research, 123, 130
quality of life, 42
quantitative research, 127

R

race, 42, 160
racism, 160
range, viii, ix, 2, 5, 7, 16, 30, 33, 35, 47, 48, 51, 55, 70, 74, 86, 90, 91, 125, 154, 156, 157, 159, 160, 161, 162
rating scale, 53, 78
ratings, 12, 78
reading, 161
reality, 61, 65
recall, 99
receptors, 28, 84, 138, 144
recognition, viii, 6, 29, 44, 49, 123
recollection, 35, 38, 123
recovery, x, 4, 22, 86, 87, 90, 95, 97, 98, 99, 100, 102, 103, 134, 149
recruiting, 34
recurrence, 28, 30, 81, 82, 84, 87, 101, 102, 144, 163
reduction, 18, 141
reforms, 65
regression, 112
regulation, 2, 7, 12, 26, 102, 137, 149
reinforcers, 21
rejection, 5, 106, 138
relapses, 79, 103
relationship, vii, viii, x, 2, 9, 16, 17, 19, 21, 22, 23, 26, 38, 42, 43, 47, 48, 52, 56, 101, 102, 105, 106, 107, 115, 117, 120, 123, 128, 145, 152, 163, 164
relationships, 9, 10, 16, 17, 18, 87, 101, 102
relatives, 60
relevance, 22, 129, 149
reliability, 88, 113, 154
remission, ix, x, 50, 73, 86, 87, 88, 89, 90, 91, 93, 94, 95, 97, 98, 99, 100, 103
replacement, 135, 145, 147
replication, 120
reproduction, 4, 8
resistance, 98
resolution, ix, 70
resources, 45, 49, 50, 51, 52, 53, 54, 55, 98, 162
responsibility, 17, 63, 123, 126
responsiveness, vii, 1, 2, 4, 5, 6, 7, 8, 11, 13, 18, 20, 25, 27, 144, 149
restructuring, 9
retrieval, 25
rights, 158
risk, vii, viii, xi, 1, 2, 4, 8, 9, 10, 11, 14, 15, 16, 17, 19, 29, 30, 31, 38, 39, 41, 42, 43, 44, 45, 48, 49, 51, 52, 53, 54, 56, 57, 61, 63, 64, 73, 74, 79, 80, 81, 84, 86, 87, 88, 97, 99, 100, 102, 110, 114, 118, 130, 131, 132, 138, 146, 147, 152, 153, 155, 161, 164
risk factors, viii, 29, 31, 41, 42, 43, 44, 49, 56, 57, 74, 80, 84, 146
rodents, 9, 26, 133, 149
role conflict, 14
routines, 15
rural population, 19, 160

S

safety, 43, 61, 63
saliva, 144
sample, x, xii, 8, 9, 10, 11, 16, 31, 32, 34, 35, 37, 41, 42, 52, 89, 91, 98, 105, 109, 110, 113, 115, 116, 117, 118, 121, 122, 123, 124, 126, 127, 128, 151, 152, 154, 160, 161, 162
Sartorius, 118, 119
satisfaction, 16, 17, 41, 42, 52, 54
Saudi Arabia, 27
scaling, 162
Scandinavia, 14
schizophrenia, 88
school, 156
scores, 10, 12, 13, 16, 31, 32, 34, 42, 70, 72, 73, 89, 108, 111, 114, 153, 156, 157, 164
search, 30, 31, 61
searching, 7, 30
secretion, 5, 7, 8, 75, 77
security, 118
selective estrogen receptor modulator, 149
self, xi, 3, 11, 12, 13, 16, 17, 18, 20, 28, 40, 41, 42, 48, 53, 60, 78, 87, 106, 108, 113, 122, 123, 126, 127, 128, 154, 158, 160, 161, 162, 164
self-efficacy, 11, 13, 17, 18, 20, 40
self-esteem, 28
self-perceptions, 106
self-reports, 87
sensitivity, 7, 9, 17, 20, 28, 31, 32, 33, 78, 79, 83, 84, 154, 161
separation, 27

serotonin, 6, 26, 75, 81, 137, 143
serum, 76, 77, 83, 145, 146, 148
services, viii, xi, 30, 34, 37, 47, 49, 53, 54, 56, 57, 63, 64, 87, 118, 122, 123, 128, 153, 155, 161
severity, ix, 2, 8, 30, 51, 59, 86, 87, 98, 100, 102, 109, 113, 114
sex, 21, 78, 114, 132
sex differences, 21
sex hormones, 78
sex steroid, 132
sheep, 5, 9, 24
side effects, 63
sites, 18, 155
skills, 51, 155
skin, 42, 147, 158
sleep disturbance, vii, 35, 98, 152
smoking, 42
sociability, 115
social care, 54
social class, 39
social context, 13
social development, x, xi, 106, 107, 108, 109, 110, 111, 112, 114, 115, 131, 132
social environment, 4, 18
social housing, 149
social infrastructure, 15
social network, 26, 42
social status, 114
social stress, 148
social support, 16, 17, 19, 24, 26, 27, 38, 39, 40, 42, 45, 49, 98, 120, 153, 164
sociocultural practices, vii, 1, 2
socioeconomic status, 27, 37, 43, 160
software, 91
South Africa, 15, 117
Spain, 85, 92, 105
species, 4, 5, 9
specificity, 31, 32, 33, 81, 101, 144, 154, 161, 163
spectrum, 51, 73, 74, 98
speech, 119
spin, 52
spousal support, 17
Sprague-Dawley rats, 137
SPSS, 91
stability, 7, 163
stages, 144
standard error, 70
stereotypes, 14
steroids, 26, 78, 133, 141, 143, 148, 149
stigma, 48, 52, 53

stimulus, 106
strain, 16, 123
strategies, viii, 30, 49, 50, 51
strength, 45
stress, vii, 1, 2, 4, 7, 10, 11, 15, 16, 17, 18, 20, 22, 24, 26, 27, 43, 52, 56, 81, 82, 83, 84, 98, 102, 120, 127, 128, 132, 133, 134, 138, 139, 141, 142, 144, 145, 146, 147, 148, 149, 153
stressful events, 19
stressful life events, 16, 49, 161
stressors, v, xi, xii, 11, 13, 16, 17, 23, 37, 38, 43, 81, 121, 123, 124, 125, 126, 127, 128, 134, 151, 161, 162
strong interaction, 75
substrates, 144
suicidal ideation, 152, 155
suicide, 34, 93, 153
suicide attempts, 34, 93
supervision, 51, 52, 55
suppression, 77, 83, 133, 136, 140, 146, 148
surveillance, 55, 56
survival, 5, 89
susceptibility, 75, 81
Sweden, 47, 49, 51, 52, 54, 57
Switzerland, 69, 165
symptom, ix, 3, 53, 70, 78, 88
symptomology, 11, 16, 17, 25, 132
symptoms, v, ix, 2, 3, 8, 11, 12, 15, 17, 27, 33, 40, 41, 42, 53, 54, 60, 61, 63, 64, 69, 70, 71, 72, 73, 74, 76, 79, 80, 81, 87, 88, 90, 95, 97, 98, 99, 101, 103, 109, 133, 135, 136, 137, 138, 145, 152, 153, 154, 156, 160, 161
synapse, 26
synaptic plasticity, 139
syndrome, ix, 28, 35, 37, 40, 46, 63, 69, 85, 107, 109, 120
synthesis, 57, 137
systems, 9, 51, 78, 137, 141, 143

T

telephone, 37
temperament, vii, 1, 11, 12, 13, 18, 20, 22, 26, 118
temperature, 147
tension, xi, 17, 121, 123, 126, 127
tertiary education, 124
testosterone, 5
test-retest reliability, 127
theory, 130, 133
therapy, 20, 50, 61, 64

threat, 5
threshold, 15, 95
threshold level, 15
thyroid, 8, 9, 23, 26, 28, 82, 98
time, v, vii, viii, ix, xi, 3, 6, 9, 13, 14, 15, 18, 20, 21, 22, 23, 28, 29, 48, 50, 51, 53, 54, 59, 60, 62, 63, 64, 69, 70, 71, 72, 73, 74, 78, 80, 83, 86, 87, 88, 91, 95, 97, 98, 100, 108, 112, 115, 119, 120, 121, 122, 123, 126, 127, 128, 134, 138, 139, 143, 144, 146, 156
time frame, 50, 127
timing, 5, 25, 102, 120
tradition, 15
training, 51, 54, 61, 63, 64
transcription, 147
transition, vii, 1, 2, 4, 13, 18, 20, 48, 51, 101, 124, 129
transition period, 4, 13
translation, 50
transmission, 164
transportation, 155
treatment methods, 98
trend, ix, 59, 137
trial, 23, 55, 61, 79, 80, 83, 118, 129
triggers, 48
tryptophan, 9, 23, 146
turnover, 6

U

UK, 49, 53, 54, 57, 69
ultrasound, 147
uncertainty, ix, 59, 63
underlying mechanisms, 137, 138
United States, viii, 2, 14, 16, 29, 57, 64
urban population, 119
urinary tract, 40, 41
urinary tract infection, 40, 41
US Department of Commerce, 46

V

Valencia, 105, 107, 118
validation, viii, 21, 29, 31, 33, 34, 52, 53, 55, 117, 155, 163
validity, 2, 81, 113, 119, 124, 127, 136, 154, 157, 161
values, 75, 125, 126, 157, 161
variability, 153, 156

variable, x, 51, 86, 106, 108, 116
variables, 16, 26, 27, 28, 37, 42, 43, 48, 64, 88, 91, 107, 108, 110, 111, 112, 116, 118, 147
variance, 17, 74
variation, 25, 70, 75, 99
varicose veins, 40, 41
vasopressin, 20, 147
violence, 160
vocational training, 156
vulnerability, 4, 10, 11, 17, 22, 50, 52, 74, 75, 77, 80, 103, 138, 160
vulnerability to depression, 11, 17, 160

W

war, 35
water, 135
weight loss, vii, 152
well-being, xii, 17, 56, 132, 142
Western countries, 48
withdrawal, ix, xi, 9, 21, 63, 69, 78, 79, 132, 134, 135, 136, 138, 140, 141, 142, 146, 148
wives, 34
women, vii, viii, ix, x, xi, xii, 2, 3, 4, 7, 8, 9, 10, 11, 13, 14, 15, 16, 17, 18, 22, 23, 24, 25, 26, 27, 29, 30, 31, 33, 34, 35, 36, 37, 38, 40, 41, 42, 44, 45, 46, 47, 48, 49, 50, 51, 52, 53, 54, 56, 57, 59, 60, 61, 63, 64, 65, 69, 70, 72, 73, 74, 75, 76, 77, 78, 79, 80, 82, 83, 85, 86, 87, 88, 89, 90, 91, 93, 94, 95, 97, 98, 99, 100, 101, 103, 105, 106, 107, 109, 110, 115, 116, 118, 121, 122, 123, 124, 125, 126, 127, 128, 129, 131, 132, 133, 134, 135, 136, 137, 138, 141, 143, 146, 147, 148, 149, 151, 152, 153, 154, 155, 156, 157, 159, 160, 161, 162, 163, 164, 165
work roles, 4
workers, 34, 77
work-related stress, xi, 121, 125, 128
World Bank, 56
worry, vii

Y

yield, 156